Embracing Willendorf:

A Witch's Way of Loving Your
Body to Health and Fitness

by

H. Byron Ballard

Smith Bridge Press
Asheville, NC

Contact author at www.myvillagewitch.com

Edited by D. A. Sarac
TheEditingPen.com

Cover Design by Susan A. McBride
susanmcbridedesign.com

Embracing Willendorf: A Witch's Way to Loving Your Body to Health and

Fitness/ H. Byron Ballard. -- 1st ed.

ISBN-10: 0-9967583-5-6
ISBN-13: 978-0-9967583-5-2

Smith Bridge Press
Asheville, NC
SmithBridgePress@gmail.com

Blessed be the strong and round girls,

with their fierce, wild hearts.

Per ardua ad Terra.

My affinity for Willendorf has grown over the past twenty-five years or so—to the extent she is my first, and so far only, tattoo. She is one of the oldest manifestations of the Great Mother and represents, for me at least, a time when women were honored. And our shapes are similar too, so identifying with her was easy! Imagine my delight, then, to read this book that twines health and healing and love of body with the earthly center of spirituality. I met Byron back in the '90s and witnessed her journey, watched as she shed pounds and gained vibrant energy, observed her rampage against the mainstream mindset of body shaming, saw how she examined the attention she received based on her size, and admired how she was constantly and faithfully loving herself through the whole of it. The genius of this book is that she teaches us how to do that too. Reading *Embracing Willendorf* is like sitting down with Byron for tea and conversation or taking one of her workshops where she simultaneously comforts and challenges us. Her conversational style is both refreshing and cozy, giving us a sense of intimacy and truthfulness, allowing her insights to inspire our own. She encourages us to interact with our own inner body through journaling, ritual, and movement. This book is about getting in touch with our bodies—and it's about unconditional love for ourselves. The time to start this process is NOW.

~Renee Robb-Cohen: A Celebration of Being

Embracing Willendorf reads like a friendly conversation with a beloved wisewoman. It is full of encouragement, gently worded suggestions, and loving advice. Ms. Ballard shares stories of her own journey to a strong, healthy body with humor and honesty. She leads us through both the triumph of fitting into coveted blue jeans and the travail of hitting a crazy-making plateau in her weight loss. There is good practical advice about exercise and meal portions and a balanced diet, intermixed with good spiritual advice about listening to your heart, setting intentions, and journaling about your experiences. *Embracing Willendorf* is a fine guidebook for the journey into loving your body and treating it well. I highly recommend it.

~Alice Rain

In *Embracing Willendorf: A Witch's Way of Loving Your Body to Health and Fitness*, Byron Ballard delivers a passionate, practical, and honest approach to loving oneself and caring for one's earthly and spiritual body. Having lived in the body of the Willendorf myself for almost thirty years, I loved the raw and beautiful candor with which Byron regales her story of self-transformation. At times it felt as if she wrote the book just for me! It left me inspired and ready, finally, to find my own place where the love of my body is greater than that of the world's judgments about it. High praise for this high priestess! Thank you, Byron, for sharing your journey with us!

~Allison Mullins

Byron Ballard's *Embracing Willendorf* is a welcome return to the home of the body temple. As a priestess of the Great Goddess, she will introduce you to "your deep earth self." She teaches radical self-love, beginning with how to stop bullying yourself by choosing one thing to unreservedly love about your body. In her friendly, conversational style, Byron offers a quick course in Pagan 101 (a little altar, a few affirmations, sitting quietly for a few minutes a day), then moves on to the idea of trusting your own body, served up with a side of self-love that might make you blush. She is a uniquely qualified stand against our body-hostile culture, so permeated with a religion of guilt and mortification of the flesh. Nondogmatic and with plenty about the pitfalls of losing weight (yes, you will miss your old shape), this may be the only "diet" book with a recipe for Cherry Yum Yum at the end, because loving yourself always means enjoying life.

~Cari Ferraro

Byron Ballard's book, *Embracing Willendorf: A Witch's Way of Loving your Body to Health and Fitness* offers tender relief from the abuse of the diet industry from page one. The book feeds the impoverished, starving mind and heart of the diet junkie with a lucid reshaping. Not for her (and us) the treacherous shaming into self-hate-fueled action. Her approach to health and wellness—with the help of the round, unashamed, earthy Venus of Willendorf as muse—asks us to trade dependence upon the illusion of diet as cure for one that promotes imperfect, delicious, rigor, and discipline around our eating choices and replaces the fear and demented self-loathing with transcendent self-love. In her delightful recounting of having eliminated sugar as a mainstay of her diet, we are treated to the story of a real woman who struggles and lands on the sanity of also eliminating objectification, faultfinding, and despair over her body to reach a truce—not a complete victory over the demon sweet. Of all the truth and wisdom in this book, her acceptance that there will be occasional chocolate or cherry yum yum strikes me as hard-won and valuable sanity. She advocates for healthy eating (the rather universal precepts of a Mediterranean-type eating style) but spares us the arrogant "my way is best" marketing baloney. And here we come to the heart of the matter: this is simply not another patriarchal take on women's bodies and how they should be. There is no male gaze. No hideous militaristic metrics for success. No starvation. No dangerous pills. No rejection. And though Byron exalts in the health and ease of her new slimmer body, it comes without that diet-club edge of idiotic preening. Here is a woman who loves herself like the Great Mother would have us love ourselves. And that changes the brain that changes the body that changes everything.

~Deirdre Morro James

Contents

ACKNOWLEDGMENTS

This book was written in 2003, shopped by an inexperienced agent who discovered it was too Pagan for the mainstream "Diet and Health" market and too "Diet and Health" for the Pagan market. It malingered in a file on my computer, and I developed a workshop from the material—a workshop that has been presented in different places across the Southeast. The years have passed, and I've maintained the original weight loss and even added another fifteen pounds to the overall number.

The editor at Smith Bridge Press (publisher of my recent Appalachian folk magic book *Asfidity and Mad-Stones*) thought we should take another look at it and consider publishing it through that delightful indie press. I rewrote and updated much of it, added a quirky suggested reading list, and sent it over to the editor.

And here it is. Some of the information in the early chapters of this book first appeared in *WNC Woman* magazine in 2003. Thanks to Julie Parker for the opportunity to share Willendorf with a select and wonderful audience.

More thanks to my author friends and mentors including MariJo Moore, Randy Russell, Janet Barrett, Charles Price, Ruth Perschbacher, Vicki Lane, Alex Bledsoe, Betty Cloer Wallace, Wayne Caldwell, Kate Laity in her various guises, and Joan Medlicott. They listened and advised and bought me coffee—and grits—thanks, Charles! My first readers were brave and crazy—Alice Rain, Cari Ferraro, Deirdre Morrow James, Allison Mullins—and terribly helpful.

Gratitude to my co-religionists—the expanding and often physically contracting Pagan community that I am privileged to play and work with throughout the US and UK.

My editor, Annie Sarac, and all the good people at Smith Bridge Press. To Susan McBride for her fineness, fierceness, and finesse.

And thanks to all the friends and acquaintances who let me tell the story of their personal embrace of Willendorf, people who came to love their earthy, juicy selves and somehow found happiness. Who knew?

FOREWORD — THE BIG LIE

Our American obsession with fitness is culture-driven, as well as fueled by a capitalist system that has to keep selling and selling. The environment is showing dramatic signs of stress, as are our credit card bills, but the only way we can save our nation is to drive the economy by purchasing things we don't need with money we don't have. And if, for some reason, you don't feel the desperate need to consume—that is the birthright of every American—we have a subculture of marketers who can make you want it. Try watching television for ten minutes at any time, day or night. How many pizza, burger, and instant-cookie commercials can you spot? How many new cars must we buy to bolster the American way of life?

Michael taught me the subtle art of pool and is my oldest friend in the world. We complained once that the last two groups of people in the world who can be mocked and ridiculed with impunity are hillbillies and fat people. We, sadly, are both and so must put up with our share of hostility from the skinny outlanders who frequent our tourist town. Neither of us has any intention of denying our deeply redneck roots, but our body masses change with interesting regularity. At this writing, both of us enjoy a degree of slimness that is, frankly, astonishing. His snap-front Western shirts reveal a shaped-up and slimmed-down torso, which I'm sure his horse appreciates on the long wagon-trail things he does. With his curly brownish hair and cheerful disposition, he is becoming a buff Cupid.

For now. All this could change in a twinkling. But for the moment he and I are safe from the ridicule of perfect strangers and hostile family members.

But that's not true for all Americans. Despite the good work of the gorgeous Melissa McCarthy and others, it is not cool to be fat. Fat teenagers are especially vulnerable, I suspect, but anyone who bulges in all the wrong places can expect to feel the wrath of our perfection-obsessed society. Although the majority of our citizens are now classified as overweight or obese, the popular culture is dominated by images of sickly thin starlets and beefy sports stars. Supermarket tabloids worry that Oprah will keel over because of her over-150 poundage, although we find it difficult to get out and take a walk in the neighborhood. Nighttime TV loves to mock the gravity challenged, and if there is such a thing as a Fat Person Anti-Defamation League, they don't get much press coverage. Social media does seem to be blooming with sites and essays about the grief engendered through fat-shaming, but as is always true, don't read the comments.

I recall one of those *Maury and Company*-type shows a few years ago that featured "men who love fat women." The women were dressed in the most unflattering, Frederick's of Hollywood sort of clothes. And the men seemed apologetic about this perversion they were admitting to on national television. But after all the hype, when they actually got down to talking, the guys seemed sincere and nice and the women cared for them too. It was necessary, though, to turn their relationships into a freak show in order to satisfy... what? Ratings? Probably. And what drives the ratings? The interest of those people sitting at home, watching something stupid and mean on TV or online to make their own lives seem less awful.

But maybe those people want to feel less freakish themselves. To feel that somewhere in the world there is someone who is nice and reasonably attractive who will love them because of, rather than in spite of, their girth.

So if it's so hard to be fat in our culture, why don't people lose weight? Why don't we simply exert our willpower and cut back on calories, get more exercise and slim down?

The reasons we don't are legion and also highly individual. Unlike some addictive substances, like alcohol and cigarettes, a fat person can't simply stop eating, quit that habit cold turkey. We need those calories to keep the machine working, after all.

And some people overeat for a variety of emotional reasons. They use food sometimes as a sedative, sometimes as a stimulant, sometimes as a way to not feel what they don't want to feel.

I used to work in a bookstore, and I saw diet book after diet book gain in popularity, sell out, be reordered, see perfectly lovely people clamoring for some way to get thinner, to be better. To be honest, I saw very few people actually follow through with their strong intentions for fitness and weight loss. Mostly, they came back a year later and bought the next hot diet book, usually hawked by someone they've seen on television, doing the ubiquitous book tour.

In the face of a culture that damns the overweight, why would anyone choose to be the object of this animosity and ridicule? Self-esteem issues aside, what is it with Americans that makes them suffer the fools who mock them? I have discovered something very interesting in this Willendorf process. I read and listen to ads for the newest miracle pill or exercise machine or diet regimen. They promise money-back, instant results. We hear from young and old folks who have lost twenty-five or fifty or one hundred twenty pounds, and their lives have changed. Woo-hoo! Remember Jared the Subway Guy before his fall from grace? Several weight-loss chains show before and after shots of local people who have lost X number of pounds and can now cavort in the surf wearing a thong. My favorite is the woman on a radio ad who wants to lose "that embarrassing pouch" at her stomach that has marked her since the birth of her child years ago.

Here's what I've discovered and believe to be true. Americans would like to be fit and healthy. They do not, however, want to change their entire lives to achieve this because, face it, they are busy people with full lives. So they look for a program, pill, or machine that will make this tedious process easy. That word is the key. Plug us into whatever it is, and let us do it along with taking the kids to school and going to work and arguing on Facebook in the evening.

So the weight-loss industry gives us pills, programs, and machines, and they assure us it's easy. Do this. It'll work and it's easy. Effortless weight loss. The big lie.

So we invest in the gym membership or the money-back-guaranteed diet pills, and we try to plug that into our already overburdened lives. And it may even work at first. We let down our defenses and dream of sitting in an airplane seat without getting pinched nerves in our thighs. We fantasize about wearing a two-piece bathing suit come summer. We let ourselves believe that this time it's going to work.

And then we fail. Life gets the better of us, we don't take time for the gym, and we can't afford more of the pills. We feel guilty that we're spending so much attention on the size of our waists when the world is going to hell in a handbasket. The weight we lost comes back, we put away the sizes-smaller clothes for the next time, and we live our lives, a little sadder maybe, a little heavier certainly.

And after a while, we won't even try those fads anymore because we always fail. We don't have the requisite willpower or guts or motivation to do this thing. We look around us at other Americans, and we see that we are not alone. Sure, we don't look like the people on awards shows or in the movies, but hey, we're not so bad. And we're not alone. Go into a mall or grocery store or golf course, and you'll see other fat Americans.

We also figure something must be badly wrong with us if we can't do this thing that everyone insists is easy. Gosh, if this is easy and I can't do it, I must be really bad. Or dumb. Or weak. It's easy, right? Then why can't I do it?

Because it's not easy.

There. I've said it. Changing your body from fat to fit is not easy, and I don't care who tells you it is. You aren't learning to eat for a month or six months. You aren't developing an exercise routine to get you to a goal. You are changing your whole entire life. It is a huge commitment, and it is not easy. You will be changing the way you perceive yourself and the way you are in the world for the rest of your life. And if you can do that, when you can do that, you are to be praised and congratulated for doing something that not everyone can do, for doing something that is very difficult. Like climbing Mount Everest. Every day for the rest of your long and happy life.

Sure, it gets easier once you've set a routine and have ways to help you stick to it. But this process is not easy. And if you think it is, you will fail again. You will be another fat American at the mall, grateful that they now make clothes in your size. And dreaming of a suit jacket that fits you across the chest, shoulders, and waist at the same time. Dreaming of being able to walk into any department except "Big and Tall" or "Plus" and buy a pair of pants.

Well, stop dreaming and start loving your body to health and fitness. No, it's not going to be easy. But I promise you, it's going to be worth it. Sure, you'll feel better and look better. But when you start listening to the magnificent thing that is your body and stop being ashamed of it and actually love the delicious skin you're in, the people around you (as well as your fine self) will reap the benefits of that joy and glow.

That's all well and good. But I suggest you be selfish. Do it for you.

INTRODUCTION

I lost seventy-five pounds in my initial weight loss. People who hadn't seen me in several months were shocked, and close friends watched my process as the incredible shrinking Byron.

And everyone wanted to know how I did it. Is it Atkins? Is it working with your blood type? All protein? Weight Watchers? How? What's the magic bullet? How did the fat woman we've always known change so drastically?

And why?

I've always been a strong advocate for large women. As a '70s-era feminist, I've often opined that the dominant culture's obsession with female slimness is a tyranny. Keep women physically small, and they are more easily intimidated, controlled, kept in their place. I remember being a strong, powerful, and fat teenager: answerable to myself, fierce and indomitable.

College brought lovers and breakups and friendships I still cherish. I leapt into my woman-years more confident than the culture said I had a right to be, perhaps because I come from a family of large women and was never chastised or humiliated by my mother or any of her family because of my weight. There was the occasional catcall or harsh comment from unknown morons on the street, but those were easily deflected by a self-loving woman who strode through the world, literally larger than life.

Each year, I gained a little weight until I hit grad school. That was a difficult, depressing time, and I discovered that when I was sad—unlike my friends—I didn't eat. I'm a stress-faster, not a stress-eater. I also lived a mile from school and didn't have a car. So I walked weight off and lost some of my *joie de vivre*. With my MFA and release from Dallas, I returned to my natural optimism, eating patterns, and lack of exercise.

In January of 2002, almost a year after my mother's death, my midwife gently but firmly suggested I have some blood work done, and a week later, the results were read to me over the phone. My blood sugar level was much too high as was my cholesterol. As I hung up the phone, I knew my life was going to change dramatically—that the years of living fat were over. I intuitively (and later with help from a nutritionist) developed a program that has worked for lowering and stabilizing my blood sugar, lowering my cholesterol and shedding happily earned pounds. I call this program "Embracing Willendorf" because I am determined to continue loving my magnificent body as it adapts to new ways of nurture as I love it to health. Gulp. And fitness.

Here I am—years later—a glowing, blissful shadow of my former self. My new body constantly amazes me. Like a new car, I keep taking her out on the road, seeing what she can do. At the beginning, I started out with a gentle walk and went on to do three brisk miles each and every morning. I do tai chi, daily, before bed. I hike in the treasured Smoky Mountains. I practice extreme gardening. Heck, I even climbed the apple tree in the backyard just to see if I could.

This is an amazing adventure, and I am thrilled to be your guide to loving your own elegant and powerful self.

Welcome to Willendorf.

CHAPTER ONE

WHO IS WILLENDORF?

We've all seen her—the Paleolithic Playboy model with pendulous breasts, enormous hips and buttocks, legs that taper to a point. Her head is a curious flat mass of curls, her face— seemingly not the most important body part of this particular Deity—is not visible. When she was discovered in 1908, those relics were found all over Old Europe (that part of Eastern Europe referred to as "New Europe" by the State Department). They were called Venuses by archaeologists and anthropologists who thought they were Stone Age pornography.

As our views of our ancestors gained sophistication, theories were promoted in which those small and ubiquitous statues were icons from a fertile age of Mother Goddess worship— "mother" goddess because the Venus figures were corpulent and proud and oh-so-obviously fertility figures. They are now generally called "figurines" or "goddesses" (small g), and she is called the Goddess of Willendorf after the Austrian town where she was found. Sometimes she's even called "Willi." She is big (though the actual piece is less than five inches long) and she is beautiful, like each of us.

The key to success in this life-changing and life-affirming program is to love your body. I mean really love it—regarding yourself in the mirror with a feeling slightly better than revulsion just won't do the trick. The barrier to this is deeply cultural. Americans live in a schizophrenic environment that honors thinness and health while producing some of the fattest people on the planet. This dichotomy is curious but clearly illustrates the problematic relationship that we have with our bodies and the food we need to fuel them.

A few years ago, I met a charming woman who was battling chronic fatigue and walked with the help of a cane. She was picking up a special order at the bookstore about the descent of Inanna, and I commented that it was a very good book that made striking use of the story of Inanna's descent to the underworld to meet her sister, Erishkegal. She said a friend had told her it could be a helpful metaphor for what she was going through in her own health crisis. This woman was obviously educated, spiritually savvy, open-minded. We talked a bit about her health, and I asked her the question I should have tattooed on my forehead—are you loving your body? The polite smile faded from her face, and she looked away. No, she finally said, I don't suppose I am. Her face was puzzled and very, very sad. How can she love this thing that encases her spirit, this thing that is causing her so much anguish? Why does her spirit have to be housed in all this... flesh? I touched her hand and expressed my opinion that the deep meditations around Inanna's descent would indeed be helpful to her, speaking as a priestess of this Sumerian Deity. She smiled again and left the store.

There are things that genetics, environment, accident, or lifestyle have done to you that are not fixable by learning to love yourself. Loving your body won't cure an incurable disease or replace an amputated limb, and it doesn't take the place of a trained healthcare professional with good diagnostic skills. I long for a few words or a special herbal concoction that will heal those ills or at least alleviate pain and other debilitating symptoms. Loving your body, even in its infirmity and illness, may help you take better care of it as it heals or—in the case of chronic illness—as you learn to cope with being differently abled.

Let me state from the outset that my worldview and philosophy are earth-centered, Pagan. I don't see my body as the barrier between the "real" me and a genuine spiritual life. My eyes are not fixed on a heavenly home that can only be achieved when the real "me"—my soul—has passed from the misery of this world. This rich and beautiful planet is all the home I need, thank you very much. It supplies all my needs and wants, and I love it dearly.

Because of my spiritual worldview, I won't deal in sin or guilt or mortification of the flesh. I simply don't believe that an angry deity has sentenced you to the humiliation of living in an uncontrollable clay suit, which you must punish to bring into conformity. You can waste a lot of good time beating yourself up about why you eat too much or don't exercise enough. You can blame it on your genes or the way you were parented or on your current partner, but if you take personal responsibility for this incredible instrument that is you, you can make amazing changes in your emotional as well as your physical well-being. Imagine waking to the sound of birdsong, luxuriating in the way your body feels in the warmth of your cozy blankets. Walking to the kitchen for a bracing gulp of cold, fresh water or spicy tea, your feet and legs taking you from bed to fridge. Imagine really experiencing your life as you love the skin you're in.

I love my body and have loved it through many sizes and shapes and levels of fitness. I am a remarkable instrument, a highly adept and adaptable tool. I belong to a hardy and clever species and am connected on a cellular level to everything else.

Lofty words, Miss B, but how do they apply to me? Even if I can acknowledge this connection, how can I love my lumpy knees or my round stomach or my wide butt? What's so lovable about any of those things? In these chapters, I'm going to give you permission to love your whole self. Not that you need anyone's permission. Consider this is a permit that is not granted by the media or the church or even your kith and kin. Those entities want to control how you feel about your body for a number of reasons. The reasons are cultural (to sell you more products in order to achieve perfection and then live forever—did I mention saving the American way?), religious (your body is a sin magnet trapped in a cesspool of degradation and must be saved by whatever means necessary in order to achieve your real home in heaven), social (you love the ocean and want to go to the beach with your family—but you can't possibly be seen on the beach looking like that), and familial (you'd be so pretty if you'd lose weight—you were such a skinny kid. Oh him, yeah, he'll eat anything, he's a bottomless pit).

By the time you finish these pages, you will have the authority to love yourself totally—to love your perfect, remarkable body to health and fitness. I won't let magazines or statistics bully you. And I won't let you bully yourself.

So today—yes, today—choose one thing about your body that you adore. Your beautiful eyes, your strong calves, your long fingers. Don't tell me there's nothing—I don't believe it. We all have that little thing we're secretly proud of, that part that keeps us from despair during the bikini days of summer. Find it. Right now.

And love it, my dear. For a whole solid week, love that place that is beautiful in your eyes. And I think you'll find when you acknowledge your love of that, you'll find other parts that pass muster. Our goal is to love it all, but it takes time to cancel out the media messages and the tinny sound of that inner, critical voice. We're going to start with the basics and work our way up to loving the whole kit and caboodle.

One tool that I have found most helpful in Willendorf and in life in general is to keep a journal. Oh yes, it's all the rage these days, which is fortunate because you can find a good, inexpensive one in your local bookstore, or you can get a cheap notebook at your local discount merchant during the horrifying Back-to-School-sale time. Either way, find a little notebook and write stuff in it. Not necessarily deep and profound stuff that will live after you and should be bequeathed to your local library. A simple little notebook where you can write your weight and your exercise schedule and the nice thing that the checkout lady said to you. Of course, if you want to buy a leather-bound, handmade paper journal and write about your lonely childhood or the way politicians make you crazy, feel free. Have at it! I enjoy looking back on the months of being Changing Woman and seeing how my attitude (as well as my bust measurement) changed.

I also kept a list of affirmations and meditations that helped me, especially in the early stages. I mostly made them up, but I also found them in some pretty surprising places. A friend had a poster on her wall with a catchy phrase that I wrote on the back of my hand. I heard a song on the radio with a line that worked for me, and I wrote that down.

There are a few quotes that I've found that make me smile or keep me going. Please develop some of your own, and use them as a tourist spot on your spiritual and physical journey.

"The Spartan body will prevail!" Barbara Sayer. This was told to me not by Barbara, who is slim and strong, but by her brother, who may be strong and is certainly as good a person as I know, but is not slim.

"Inside myself is a place where I live all alone, and that's where you renew your springs that never dry up." Pearl S. Buck. This quote came from another friend, one who took one of the Willendorf workshops.

And *"i found god in myself and i loved her i loved her fiercely."* Ntozake Shange. What can I say? I am a child of my generation. This came from a cool poster on someone's Facebook wall.

Setting up an altar or meditation table as a focus for your transformational work may also be helpful. No, you don't have to order a copy of our girl Willi and set her up on an ebony table (though that would look very pretty). Find a place in your home with a flat surface—a table, the back of the toilet, the shelf above your computer monitor. Find a few things that you already own that are small, portable, meaningful, beautiful. If you want to put an antique hankie or a hand-woven place mat down as a cloth, that would be lovely. Get a candle (flame or electric) in a votive cup and arrange all the things in a way that is pleasing to your eye. You might add a small hand mirror if your chosen part isn't visible without one.

Spend a little time—a couple of minutes—looking at this beauty every day. Speak your affirmation and intention into this holy space. Dedicate some of the precious time out of your busy day to honor your reconnection with your gorgeous body. Spend moments in silence listening to what your body needs. This seems easy, but it's not: you will feel uncomfortable in it at first. The silence. You'll feel like you need to do something, anything. That you're wasting time, getting nothing done. Spending time with yourself is one of the best presents you can get and give, but most of us are so unused to being alone and tending to silence that the very process is fraught with tension and, for some, fear. You may have to nurse it along, one minute at a time, until you can work up to spending five minutes alone in silence.

See how silly that sounds? Like you, a grown person, couldn't spend five minutes sitting still and being quiet. You can, you know. I promise you it's worth the effort of adjusting to a new way of being. You'll think thoughts and feel feelings you never would have experienced otherwise.

And you'll come to know someone who is loving, generous, funny, smart, and intuitive.

You.

JOURNAL NOTES

CHAPTER TWO

Pagan Deities

Many modern Pagans—both women and men—are abundant in their physicality. It always amuses me to see depictions of the Wiccan "Lord and Lady" in which the Goddess is portrayed as a slight, delicate girl with an oddly enormous chest, protected by the equally fit and trim "Lord," a broad-shouldered Cernunnos with a muscular torso and powerful thighs.

Please. Has the artist ever been to a Pagan gathering where you can find large, powerfully round women and consorts of the pale and slim or ruddy and round variety? If this is the ideal for deity, is it also what Pagans dream of being themselves? Why?

I have some objections theologically about images of a defenseless goddess and her hunky consort, but I'm concerned here with the disconnect between us and our notions of deity. What does this set up for the Pagan community, this disconnect? Have we allowed a dominant culture to define our goddesses and gods so that a woman's razor can be successfully advertised under the name Venus, showing slim, hairless legs instead of the ripe abundance of the Roman goddess of love? Where are the hips and pendulous breasts of those earliest Venuses? The Paleolithic goddess figures that our ancestors created bear little resemblance to modern renderings of goddesses, images used to hawk products that only serve to remove us further from the natural beauty and utility of our magnificent selves.

So we are stuck with a bothersome question—do we create art that reflects our own physicality, or do we seek an ideal in our quest to portray a material representation of a spiritual being?

Even in a community of people who honor the planet as the sacred body of the divine, even among people who practice so-called earth religions, there is this peculiar notion that we must deny what we believe and are for some notion of beauty that by any standards is very modern and probably not very healthy.

So we hate our bodies. We're told that they are dirty, so we must perfume them. They are lumpy and unmuscled, so we must buy a membership at the gym or an expensive machine that will clutter up the living room and end up as a magazine rack or clothes hamper. As our strong genes allow us to live longer, fuller lives, we must erase the signs of this triumph by injecting poisons to deaden the nerves in our faces.

Is anyone else bothered by the thought of someone injecting botulism into your face so that you look younger? That they sell this product with a charming name that ends in "tox"? Are we so desperate to look younger that we willingly allow—and pay for—poisons to be pumped into our bodies?

Apparently so. Apparently it is not enough to have a surgeon nip and tuck your wrinkles away or suck the excess fat out of your body. What in the world is happening to us as a species? How can we hate ourselves so much that nothing we can do—ever—is enough to make us perfect or even acceptable? Even our teeth can no longer be merely cavity-free. They must be straightened or capped or whitened. Why? Why isn't it enough to be strong and healthy?

When even the Pagan community is not in touch with their bodies, how can there be hope for the dominant culture, which often equates "earthly" with evil and seems afraid to look their ancestors in the eye when they cross the Veil? When our own community refuses to take personal responsibility for their own bodies, why should the larger culture pay any attention to us when we talk about politics or civil liberties or environmental justice? We are Earth's first line of defense within our species, and we are no better about loving our bodies that anyone else.

Older Pagans will remember the days—inspired by the free-love hippie movements—when we cavorted in the woods on Beltane, when we raised energy through sex in rites that are variously called the Great Rite or sex magic. I came of age sexually in this golden time before

HIV/AIDS and after the Pill and Roe. Times are different now, but I am determined to remind my co-religionists of the beauties of expressed pleasure. (Chapter Fifteen is about that very thing.) Pagan culture has been clamped down by the struggles of the larger culture, to our detriment.

But I think we are beginning to change that. I have hope for my community and hope for the American community. I think we have what it takes to break out of this cycle of self-loathing and find ourselves in a world in which we love our bodies, listen to them, and do what is best for them.

I love round and voluptuous bodies. I also love long, slim ones. We are different people with different body styles. Each one perfectly beautiful. Are you still loving that favorite part? Don't forget.

JOURNAL NOTES

CHAPTER THREE

LOVING YOUR BUTT

I have an exceptionally perfect nose. No really, I do. There was a boy in high school named Sam who said he'd marry the first woman he met with a perfect nose and perfect toes. My tree-climbing, summer-barefoot, crooked long toes would not pass muster. But the nose was ideal. Not too long, not too short, just right. The kind of nose people spend thousands of dollars to achieve. But do I appreciate it? Probably not. It holds up my glasses, gets clogged during pollen season, sunburns easily. My perfect nose— I hardly notice it, unless it's causing problems.

My point in all this nose reverie is that it's not usually the perfect part that we are drawn to. It's a part or an expression or a gesture that reconnects us with our deep selves. I love my knobby knees, scarred though they are, because they look like my grandmother's. When I can get to that sweet spot, I love the upper arm sag— though I confess I'm working with weights to minimize it—because it reminds me of sleeveless polyester "shells" (remember those?) and my cousin Evvie's arms.

Over the years, you have no doubt found some body parts you love—some of you have found several. Excellent. What is it exactly you love about those parts? Are they perfect? Acceptable in the culture? Do those juicy calves always get you noticed—favorably? I promise we won't do a lot of head-focused analyzing, but we will do a little search for this because it's important in how we view all the "parts" and how we remember ourselves into a whole, vibrant person.

Think about those parts for a moment. Indulge yourself in a little nose reverie of your own. What is it about your part? Why this one above all the others? Take a moment for meditation on this because the answer may well surprise you.

Since this journey began, I've had so many positive responses to this Willendorf adventure that I want to share a few of them. Some of you have given me some fairly intimate details about your bodies—er, thanks. I, in turn, have been impossibly cheerful about some of your parts. I hope you'll all endure my enthusiasm with good grace and patience. Poor Julie was greeted with "What's your part, girl?" on several occasions. Hands, she decided, and they really are beautiful.

My old friend Sandy, who had recently returned to my life after a decade-long absence, carefully explained that she thought it was important to love herself from the inside out. I heartily concurred but still badgered her for a part.

Just one. Something she felt was extraordinary and lovely, something she could show off. Sandy thought hard about it and decided she loves her eyes. And you know what this darling girl did? She arranged to get new glasses so her eyes could do their job a little more easily. Good, sensible.

But this is the part I love. She also starting messing around with makeup. Eye shadow, mascara, brow pencil. The next time I saw her she was quite pleased with herself. She wasn't doing this because she saw it in a magazine or because she wanted a man to notice her (though both of those may also be true). She did it because she found a body part that she loved without reservation, and once she fell in love, she wanted to show it off. She did the healthy thing—new spectacles. But she also did the fun thing— makeup. Atta girl!

Now that you've done the right thing and claimed a portion that is exquisite, powerful, unique, I want more from you. You knew that was coming, didn't you? I want you to apply this sense of unparalleled devotion to other special parts. Give yourself carte blanche to love all the great, good, pretty good, and okay parts of your splendid body. Spend a week doing that— nodding to yourself in mirrors as you recognize the investment you've made in all those grand parts. You don't have to go out and buy a ruby ring for the lovely hands that you now cherish and appreciate, but you could put on a little lotion after you wash the dishes. It's not strictly necessary to have an expensive facial at a local day spa but you could whip up some egg white and try a homemade masque, maybe putting some cucumber slices on your eyes.

When someone mentions your eyes or hands or hair—and they will—practice being your gracious self. No need to tell them every detail of your Willendorf embrace. Just thank them and smile. It works like a charm, if you'll pardon the expression.

So you've spent two weeks going from the easy-to-love part to the trickier bits. Yes, I have thick, sturdy ankles, peasant girl that I am. They are powerful, strong, and in that, they are beautiful. Doesn't matter what the romance novels say. And they are dead sexy in thick cotton socks and hiking boots. Yes, you've acknowledged, your shoulders are too slender to play football, but you are a good spelunker and never get that claustrophobic trapped feeling when exploring your favorite caves. See? You've begun loving those bits as well. Good for you. Are you smiling a little bit more? Or are you waiting for Willendorf to lower the boom?

Consider it lowered. Now comes the hard part. Courage, my friends.

I want you to take a part—for me, I will confess, it was my large, bodacious, Hottentot butt—that you find difficult to acknowledge, much less love. You picked out a favorite part. Now I want you to rise up to the challenge of the difficult bits. You can do this. I know you can. We'll do this hard part together. It'll surprise you. I know it surprised me.

JOURNAL NOTES

CHAPTER FOUR

I was in high school when I first heard about the "Hottentot Venus." She was an African woman of the Khoisan people named Sarah (Saartjie) Baartman. Baartman was abducted in 1810 and exhibited in England and France to great acclaim. Barbara Chase-Riboud did careful research and has written a sensitive and enraging book called *The Hottentot Venus* that I was fortunate to read as I was working this program. Baartman came back into public consciousness when her remains were finally returned to her African homeland in 2002 and finally buried in her native land after nearly 200 years in Europe.

Baartman was known for her extremely large buttocks and hips—a condition called steatopygia—and she was exhibited with other "freaks" and curiosities to take advantage of the voracious European tastes for oddities. You will appreciate the delicious irony of a culture that was soon to force its own women into corsets and butt-enhancing bustles and still paid good money to ogle, torment, and brutalize an African woman who had those accouterments naturally. Baartman died at the age of twenty-five in France, and her body was dissected by Napoleon's pet surgeon. Her brain, genitals, and articulated skeleton were exhibited in France until 1985.

She was victimized for nearly two centuries, but she and her big behind were my high school heroes. In that long-ago time, we didn't know much about Baartman—I didn't even know her name until Chase-Riboud's book. I had no idea of her origins or her degradation or her eventual death in Paris at such a tender age. All I knew was that she had a protruding butt, just like mine. Well, to be honest, I never was quite so well-endowed, but it certainly felt that way to me sometimes. I was just another freak.

As an Anglo-Celt woman spectacularly endowed in the cheeks department, I felt a deep kinship with the Venus. I lugged this pointed posterior around at the back of my body no matter what I did. Diet and exercise didn't seem to faze it—my top and legs would get smaller, but my hips were undeterred. At my first college theatre audition, I was careful to wear dark pants and a lighter shirt—the camouflage that I had developed over the years. Another actor said to me afterward—your reading was really good, but you looked kind of weird with that tiny top and great big hips. How gratifying it was to hear that.

That may be the most surprising thing about my body change during this year of Willi. I look at myself sideways in mirrors and ponder what once would have been my silhouette, and it's totally different. I don't know if it's the combination of diet and exercise, or if it is somehow age related, but my body is very different. So different, in fact, that there came a point where I lost my sense of balance. I no longer had my lifelong anchor balancing me to the back. It took a couple of weeks for my body to recalibrate, during which time I sometimes fell over while walking. I spent those weeks walking with my legs far apart and being overly conscious of gravity. It worked though. It is very strange for me to not think of myself as a woman with a big butt. But I am. After all these years, that is not a defining characteristic of my appearance.

So what's your "big butt"? Is it fat thighs or crooked teeth? Is it big feet or thick ankles? Male-pattern baldness? What's that part that makes you cringe to think of it—much less look at it? "You would be such a pretty girl/handsome guy, if only you..." What fills in that blank for you?

Deal with it right now. Yeah, it's painful, but it's been painful all those years, and we're going to deal with it right here, right now. Once and for all.

We're going to begin with a guided meditation. I will be your guide into the labyrinth of parts. Remember, it's a labyrinth, not a maze. We will follow the path to the center and retrace ourselves until we reach the outer boundaries again. This is not a trap, and there is no way to get lost. This is a pop quiz in which all sincere answers are the right ones.

Guided meditations are best experienced when you give yourself plenty of time to go through the process and plenty of time to process the experience at the end. So pick a time when you have an hour—yes, a whole hour—to devote to the exercise.

Put on something comfortable—sweatpants or a caftan or absolutely buck-naked, if that's comfortable for you. Find a place in your home where you can be undisturbed for the time of your meditation. For some of you this will be the hardest thing to manage. Can you invest in one hour to begin to undo the self-hate and loathing you've felt your whole life? Yes, I think you can. Give yourself the gift of this time. Listen to the deep, sexy voice of your own self. Remember all those beloved and okay and dreadful parts that make up the wonderful machine that is you.

Go to the bathroom and squeeze out every last drop. I have learned from personal experience that journeying on any level cannot successfully take place with a full bladder. Turn on the answering machine, turn off your cell phone. Put the dog and cats in another room or outside. Light some incense if that puts you in a proper frame of mind.

Put on some soothing music—whether New Age instrumentals or Led Zeppelin—background music that won't distract you from the journey but will give you a subliminal sense of well-being and safety. And now we will boldly go across the wine-dark seas.

CRSO

Lie on the floor in a comfortable position. For most folks, that means on your back, with possibly a small pillow under your head and another under your knees. If you are easily chilled or doing this exercise in cold weather, you might want a blanket on your legs or nearby. Put your hands on your belly and breathe deeply, feeling your belly rise and fall with each breath. Concentrate on the breathing, and close your eyes.

Imagine yourself lying on thick grass in a warm and sunny meadow. Dark clouds come across the sky and block the rays of the sun on your body. Starting with your feet, imagine the clouds uncovering the light of the sun, and the warm light falls on your body, working its way up from the soles of your feet to the top of your head. Be specific and take your time, wiggle each part as the warmth and light strike it.

Like this—the sunlight touches your big, flat feet. You breathe in, wiggling your toes. You breathe in the beauty and warmth of the sun into this part of your body. As the light warms your feet, see their beauty, their utility, their strength. Flex those babies. Feel the power.

When you have loved and appreciated and breathed your way into harmony with a particular part, let the sun shine on the next part. Yoo-hoo, thick ankles! It's me—the person you carry around all day long. Let the breathing support you as the light and warmth travel up your body. Rotate your ankles, flex your calves, bend your knobby knees, pat the jiggly flesh on your juicy thighs. Work your way slowly and inexorably up your strong, beautiful, passionate frame until you arrive at your face.

Now take your hands away from your diaphragm and rub them briskly together until they are warm from friction. Place your warm hands over your face and breathe deeply. Feel the warmth seeping into your face, into your muscles and bones and right into your sparkling and marvelous brain. Move the hands to the top of your head and imagine the warmth and light illuminating your entire body and all its parts. With light touching every part of you, remember yourself into the whole animal that you are. Let the light shine out from you, giving you a golden halo that encompasses all of you. All of you. Complete. Beautiful.

Ritual of Naming

Seven is a powerful number in many cultures, and we're going to hitch on to its power for this exercise. Every day for seven days, give yourself the gift of ten minutes in your day to do this exercise. If it helps you to record it and let it talk you through, do that.

At the end of the seven days, give yourself a naming ritual. A naming ritual can be elaborate or simple. Close your eyes and breathe. Everything we do starts in this quiet place of peace, have you realized that? Regard your remembered self in the eye of your soul and love it, respect it. Ask that self for a name that reflects the powerful and radical act you have just committed—the act of loving and healing your body, embracing the Willendorf power that resides within each of us and claiming it as your birthright. Don't worry that the name sounds silly or is too long or can't be spelled. It is your name and not another living soul need ever know it. Let the name come to your consciousness from that bright spark in your deep self. You'll know it when you hear it. I promise. Then light a candle at your altar, write your new name on a piece of paper, make yourself the gift of this whole self.

This is a good place for a journal entry. Write down your feelings and thoughts related to this event. Was it a radical act for you? Or did it seem like coming home at long last, like Odysseus? If it is more meaningful for you to draw your entry, do that. This is the beginning of all the changes, and I have found it very helpful to go back to this point of reference occasionally and feel the ecstasy of this moment. You might even mark it on your calendar, like a special birthday.

In Chase-Riboud's book, Sarah Baartman honored her feminine nature not by reveling in the juicy bounty of her hips and buttocks but in acknowledging the beauty of her small perfect hands. I don't know if this is an invention of the author's or historical fact, but in Paris and London, Saartjie frequents the shops of glovers and has dozens of pairs of red gloves made to show off this point of pride for a woman who was in exile from her land, her people and, it seems, herself. And when her remains were at last returned to South Africa in 2002, the tribal women who met the plane on the tarmac all wore red gloves in her honor. Those acts of beauty were Saartjie's naming ritual, and the soul-daughters who came after her took on the name of this beloved and much-tormented ancestor by simply wearing those gloves. How startling it must have been to look out from the doorway of the plane and see a sea of women in gloves, come to welcome their mother home. And how moving and profound. Time now to do the same for you. Go ahead and welcome yourself home.

JOURNAL NOTES

CHAPTER FIVE

Radical Self-Care

No more guilt about this, not now, not ever. Indulging in guilt makes us feel like we're doing something about a problem when really we're only feeling something about a problem. But the feeling is so heavy and so active in our roiling souls that it tricks us into thinking we're working. We aren't. We're letting old rules guide us and old triggers tell us what we should be doing.

Guilt is a way to sabotage our best intentions too. You can't do this for yourself because there are hungry children without school supplies who live in dangerous public housing. So easy to focus on that, isn't it? You'll make a little list to go by the discount store and pick up crayons, tissues, and a backpack. Maybe you'll do a Google search on child poverty in your county and sit, appalled, at the figures. Appalled and absolutely helpless.

Don't give in. It's a trap of your own devising.

I like to tell the following story with a great deal of hand waving. You'll have to imagine that and wait until we see each other at some function or festival to get the full effect. Until then, I will attempt to paint you a word picture.

You are seated, at last, on a plane, traveling with your little one or your old mom. Everyone is settling in and stowing baggage and complaining about TSA screenings. The flight attendant moves to the front of the plane as the explanation of everything begins. There may also be a film that illustrates all the important points.

She gets to the section on turbulence and tells you that there might be a loss of oxygen in the cabin, but please don't worry. If that should happen, a little mask on a tube will drop from the ceiling. You put that on and Bob's yer uncle. And—ugh, here it comes—if you are traveling with a child or elderly person, put your mask on before assisting them with theirs.

No way! we exclaim. Baby (or Mom) first! Then I will struggle along with just a little brain damage, but my loved ones will be safe.

This entire book is about loving yourself enough to tend to your physical needs, so please bear with me as I insist that you take care of you first, for once. This time when the oxygen mask falls, do the smart thing for yourself as well as all those around you—put your mask on first.

I use a *well* metaphor. Try it on for size.

The people who inhabit your intimate (and sometimes not so intimate) world soon discover that you are a good listener, a fix-it maven, an earth mother who will nurture, a fighter who loves underdogs, or all the above. They will descend on you, genuinely needing your help, your good attention.

This will go on through good times and bad. Mostly you will be willing to help—especially those people for whom you feel real affection—even when it is inconvenient or difficult for you.

As you grow more experienced in the world, you will learn to set boundaries around your time and your person. But before that happens, the essence of you—which I liken to a well of cool, sweet water—will be dipped into by all sorts of needy people.

At first the requests for water are infrequent, and the well has time to refill between encounters. But eventually the emptying will occur at ever-increasing intervals and the water level will begin to drop. If you don't find a way to curtail all this water extraction, the level won't get to replenish.

Even when you are in need yourself—for support, friendship, encouragement—the level continues to drop because your own needs are unmet. Sometimes people are careless, sometimes they are in constant crisis, sometimes they are too completely self-focused to know what's going on with you. And some people, to be honest, are users who really don't care what's going on with you because they see their need as greater and their person more important. It should go without saying that you don't need those people in your life even if they are family.

It's such an important lesson for all of us to learn, and often we have to learn it again and again. You can love someone—you can even love someone unconditionally—and still not be able to remain in a relationship with them. This is true, and I invite you to consider it.

If you haven't put a stop to the constant drain on your inner resources, on your energy and your time, there will come a day when you are empty and the well is dry. Dry as a bone. Your own needs and those of your nearest and dearest must go unmet because there is nothing left. It may take you months to refill that precious well, and for some people it never refills completely again.

Put your mask on. We are living in trying times, in challenging times. Using this program—or any program that works for you—to pay attention to and love your body will help you to honor yourself enough to say no, to let the well refill. To put on your mask first.

This is hard stuff, and I don't expect people can do it immediately. I couldn't. I still struggle with it. (But if you can, do.) Allow me to share some things you can do when you are overwhelmed by the needs of others and are working on consistently saying no and taking care of yourself.

Ten Little Things to Do as You Find Yourself Drowning in Other People's Stormy Waters

1. Pick Three

Instead of trying to solve everything that is wrong in your community or in the world, pick three things and do something real about them. What are the three issues that you are most passionate about? Those three. Let someone else take care of everything else.

2. Take a Social Media Break

Stop listening to the news, and remove yourself from social media. For three days—longer if you can. In lieu of that, stop following people who only post depressing or infuriating stuff. Disappear them. Feel no regret. If you want to catch up, you can go to their page or feed and see how they are.

3. Say No to the Things You Really, Really Don't Want to Do

You get asked to do a lot of things. Before you answer, take a moment to decide whether it is something that you want to do. Did your stomach clench at the thought of it? Say no. You can say that in whatever way works for you. "Thank you so much for that honor, but my plate is too full right now." "That is so kind! Thank you! Now is simply not a good time though. Raincheck?" Find a phrase that works for you, and memorize it so you're not fumbling around when the time comes. Let your "no"—whatever form it takes—roll trippingly off the tongue with all the sincerity you can muster.

4. Go Outside—Woods, Shore, Prairie, Mountain

Get away from the house and workplace and get outside. Park or greenway, if you're in the city. Out under the sky, if you're blessed to live in a rural place. Being in the bigness of nature has a way of settling our scratchy nerves.

5. Analyze Motivations: Yours and Theirs

It's usually easy to figure out why people want what they want from you. You're an easy mark, and they need the fix. But why do you keep saying yes? Because it gains you status? You feel better about your perceived inadequacies? You're a people-pleaser who is afraid you are unlikeable? Once you find your own reasons for always getting jammed up, it will be easier to own your own stuff and refer back to Item 3.

6. Take an Art or Craft Break

Idle hands are the devil's workshop. Schedule some playtime—either alone or with friends—and make something. Decorate some greenware. Draw a picture. Get an adult coloring book and some color-rich pencils. Practice that musical instrument that has been in its case for a decade. You get the picture—use your hands in the sacred act of creation.

7. Light a Candle

Get one of those stout seven-day candles and let it carry the stuff you can't. Imbue that pillar of wax with the grief or worry you don't need to carry, and it will make a comforting little light to guide your way to letting other people's stuff drop by your side. You are not the ghost of Jacob Marley—cut some of those heavy chains loose.

8. Put Two Needy Folks Together

You heard me. Figure out the two biggest whiners, and find a way to put them together to help each other out.

9. Scream and/or Laugh

Go stand beside a grade-level crossing at a railroad track, and when the train blows its damned horn, scream to your heart's content. You can also do this in the car. Sing along with loud rock music or better, opera. Go to a comedy club and laugh until you wet your pants.

10. Be Around People for Fun and Not to Help Out

Instead of waiting until someone is in a crisis to pay a visit, consider the people in your life that you like to spend time with and do it. Not because they need you, but because you want to. Go sit on their porch and sing while they practice their rusty guitar. Agree to meet in a park for a walk. Get coffee or a cuppa tea. Because you like them. Because you love them. Because you want to.

This might be a good place for a bit of journaling, dear friend.

JOURNAL NOTES

CHAPTER SIX

WHAT IS YOUR INTENTION?

"Just because you've got to eat, doesn't mean you've got to eat crap."

~Lobo's Deli, Athens, Georgia

What are you doing? People ask me this when they see my appearance—the "new" me. Today I went by the bookstore to pick up a special order and ran into my political junkie friend who organizes events there and coordinated the launch party for my last book. We hadn't seen each other in a bit. I was wearing my big ugly green shirt and leggings, hardly fitted clothing. She saw me and came around the counter for a fierce hug.

"Damn, woman, look at you!" she muttered in my ear. "What have you been doing?"

"Writing, a little traveling."

She grinned and pinched my arm. "No. I mean what have you done to lose more weight?"

I outlined what I'd been doing and smiled that I hadn't realized what she was really asking.

Some people, however, don't mention the change. In this age of traumatic illness, a weight loss can be the sign of something too challenging to speak of casually. One woman who has herself lost many pounds due to catastrophic illness was hesitant to say anything. She finally broached the subject very carefully and told me she'd been overweight her whole life and knew how people can be careless with their words. Her question was the best so far—is it intentional?

Isn't that lovely? She didn't make assumptions that I'd finally given in to the mountain of cultural pressure to be a size ten or that, conversely, I might be gravely ill. Is it intentional? In witchy and Pagan circles, we often speak of setting our intentions, of using magic in ways that are deeply intentional to ensure the outcomes we seek. As you begin to embrace the glory of your body, let it be intentional for you too. Be intent on flying in the face of the pervasive culture and loving your fat/skinny/short/tall body. Loving you, exactly the way you are. Right now. Do it right now.

Ouch. How did that feel? Did it seem silly? Did it seem impossible? Did it seem... wrong? That's part of the baggage we must bear in Western culture, that somehow loving ourselves is immoral, that it goes against some ancient spiritual law. Surely I should expend some energy loving others? Isn't it wrong to love yourself? Aren't there rules against it? As we discussed in the self-care chapter, you can best tend these when you yourself are healthy, focused, relaxed.

Yes, there are deeply ingrained and body-hostile rules against loving yourself. We are taught early and often that self-obsessed and arrogant people who are in love with themselves are bad role models. And that's true. Selfish, monomaniacal people who are not reflective about life are not a pretty sight, and they don't contribute much to the cultural or spiritual life of the planet.

That's not what I'm talking about. You are not that person and will not morph into that person simply because you don't hate yourself every waking moment. Yes, hate yourself. People do that, I've discovered. People who are kind to children and animals, who do good works in the community, who take care of their kith and kin. Some of those people carry around the heavy backpack of self-hate. And they've carried it around for so long that they've grown accustomed to it. I say—take that pack off and stay awhile. Have some cool spring water up here on the porch, and leave that burden be.

It is indeed okay to love yourself. There, I gave you permission. Not that you need that from me. Now—and this may be much more difficult—I want you to give yourself permission. If you are too shy or damaged or freaked out to love yourself at this moment in time, start with liking. Can you like yourself a little more? Can you begin to see yourself as someone you could talk to in line at the grocery store or the bank? Some people think more highly of that nice teller at the bank than they do of themselves. It's easier to like someone you don't interact with every minute of the day—that's a given. Try liking yourself—liking your sense of humor and your kindness and your zest for living. I think when you've grown accustomed to thinking of yourself as likable, you'll find that being lovable is just around the corner. It's a matter of intention.

I've used this guided meditation with several intentions, and I hope it works for you as well.

ଓ୫୭

Do all the aforementioned preparations for a meditation. When you are on your back, breathing deeply, comfortable, imagine yourself on a large flat rock, high about a green gorge.

Feel the warmth of the rock at your back and the warmth of the sun on your front. Warmth. You stretch and rise, walking to the edge of the rock to look into the river far below. Breathe. There is a strong rope at the edge, and you grasp it, slowly lowering yourself into the gorge below. Feel the wind on your face and your hands, arms and shoulders easily support your weight as you come down the rope and stop at the edge of the river, on a strip of sandy beach.

Behind you is a cave going into the heart of the mountain. Step inside, leaving the sun and warmth and greenness behind you. Breathe. The sounds of the river are loud in your ears and grow dim as you walk deeper into the cave. There is a shaft of sunlight that illuminates the passageway, and you follow it, going ever deeper into the mountain. The air around you is cool and damp, a welcome change from the heat and sun outside. Feel the cool air, breathe in the moisture. Your legs are strong and your body balanced as you move forward. Feel your back straightening, your breathing becoming deep and rhythmic as you walk. The cave holds no fear for you. The darkness around you is velvet and beautiful.

There is a bend in the stone, and you reach out and touch the wall beside you. Feel the coolness and smoothness of the stone. Imagine that it has worn smooth from the hands of the people who have come here before you since long ago. Breathe. As you turn the corner, the light is lost, but ahead of you a shaft of light pours in through a crack in the stone of the mountain, and it shines on something that reflects the light, multiplying the effect. You step toward this, feeling the small stones and sand beneath your feet. As you come closer, you realize it is a stone basin of rainwater that acts as a mirror for the light.

Breathe.

There is joy in this deep place and barely contained excitement. You know that the basin holds a treasure more beautiful than you can imagine. You step forward quickly, anxious to see what it holds. Breathe. As you lean forward, the secret is revealed, and you behold your own reflection in the water. The light multiplies the effect, and you see yourself as whole and remarkable. You smile as you realize that the treasure you've been seeking is this—and feel the love that is multiplying all around you, like the light.

When you are ready, come back down the tunnel and into the green and noisy world beside the river. Hoist yourself up the rope with your strong arms and shoulders and stretch out again on the warm rock. Feel the warmth permeating your body as you breathe in.

Now stretch and open your eyes. Take up your journal and write or draw how this feels for you to find the treasure in your reflection. Make a note of your intention to treat yourself like a treasure, to honor the machine that is your elegant body.

CRSO

Those were my intentions—to get my blood sugar to an acceptable level and my cholesterol under control. My plan for doing this includes watching carbohydrates. Yes, it is popular to the point of faddishness right now, but in working with a nutritionist, I've discovered that limiting carbs works for my body and my level of activity. But I do eat carbs—one hundred grams each day. I concentrate them in fresh fruits and vegetables with some whole grains. I've had to limit portions of my favorite breakfast—oatmeal. But I still eat it and love it.

Water—lots of it. Clean, filtered water is what I drink most (I keep a gallon container in the fridge), but I also love cold spring water. My friend Bonnie drinks a gallon of water a day, but I manage to do a little over the minimum daily requirement of eight eight-ounce glasses. I carry a water bottle everywhere and drink all I can. It's my beverage of choice in most situations. The occasional draft Guinness or glass of Chateau Neuf de Pape is also quite welcome.

Your body needs hydration to do its work. You know that. Plain water is best and easiest on the organs. Avoid soda—especially diet ones!—and limit your intake of caffeine if you can. That's hard for you coffee achievers, I know. But notice I said "limit," not eradicate. Hey, I'm not a monster.

Drastically reduce your use of refined sugar. Eliminate it from your diet if you can, with the possible exception of dark chocolate. This was the hardest thing I did, and I did it cold turkey when I found out my blood sugar was high. Now diabetes educators will tell you that eating too much sugar doesn't cause high blood sugar, but I wasn't taking any chances. I weaned myself from my excessive sugar intake by eating fresh fruits like apples and grapes. But the most important thing in that process was dried fruit—specifically dates and figs (both Mission and Calimyrna). They satisfy my sweet tooth (or should I say teeth?) and are very nutritious. They saved me from my heavy candy habit.

As a non-caffeinated woman in a caffeinated world, I used candy as a pick-me-up anytime my remarkable energy flagged. Midmorning, midafternoon, anytime. I walked around all day blissed out on refined sugar. Empty calories, sure, but what an effect. So the hardest thing I did was cut it out of my diet. I confess I am little afraid of it. Afraid that one bite of birthday cake will send me over the edge and I'll eat the whole damned thing.

So I avoided sugar for a long, long time. But I recently added the occasional dark chocolate square to my diet. It tastes oh so good. And I find I can limit my intake without having to think too much about it. I don't have the urge to buy a bag of Mounds bars and eat them in the car as I'm going down the road. Okay, that's a lie. I do sometimes have the urge to do it, but I don't. I eat some fresh dates instead. Or I drink more water.

The first Hallowe'en I encountered while working with Willi was much harder than I would have ever thought. Hallowe'en is a convenient excuse for everyone to eat lots of mind-altering sugary treats. There are bowls of candy everywhere—at the bank, the Red Cross, the auto mechanic's waiting room. Tiny Tootsie Rolls, Jolly Ranchers (which I despise but looked strangely delicious to my sugar-deprived brain), chocolate Kisses—they were everywhere. There was no escaping it.

The grocery store, the drugstore, the discount store—each one had shelf after shelf of large bags of cheap candy. Irresistible prices, tiny bites of perfect heaven. I thought I would lose my mind. Talk about visions of sugar plums.

I knew this would be much harder than avoiding birthday cake. I was feeling pretty cocky about my exercise routine, about the way my silhouette was shaping up, about my ability to process healthy food into lean muscles and boundless energy. Maybe I could eat a little Mounds bar, maybe I could eat a tiny KitKat bar, maybe...

No. I listened to my deep self, past the chocolate lust and the craving for crunchy sugary bites of bliss. I listened to the part of me that felt better with sugar out of my system. And yes, I listened to the tiny, frightened voice that said I still wasn't ready to risk it, to risk all that I'd done. I listened and brainstormed options for going underground or leaving the country to go someplace that didn't do trick-or-treating.

Here's what I came up with, the same technique that got me off big sugar in those early weeks. I went to a local gourmet store and bought an enormous quantity of fresh dates, and I carried them with me everywhere I went during the week before Hallowe'en. I ate them slowly with great delight. Sometimes I ate one or two, sometimes I ate a handful.

My weight didn't change appreciably, and my blood sugar levels were fine. I made it through the dangerous, vulnerable time by listening to my deep self and forming a strategy that worked for me. I did my best not to panic and to be strong.

This technique worked again almost a month later when I had my first Thanksgiving since Willendorf with my Italian-American in-laws in Atlanta. My journal for those days records five-mile forced marches every morning, floor exercise sometimes twice during the day, and forays to the local grocery store for cheese and whole bread. My in-laws, especially my sister-in-law Maria, cheerfully accepted my looks of wonder and my mad scramble for the organic peanut butter and dates every time we sat down for a meal.

It may be a stereotype, I don't know. But the women in my husband's family are great cooks, and Italian-Americans love to eat, at least in my experience. Let me tell you about the close encounter with dessert following the carb-heavy bounty of Thanksgiving dinner.

Homemade macadamia nut cookies—the scent while baking had nearly maddened me the day before—were stacked high. A plain cheesecake with a sponge cake crust stood sentinel beside it. There was a plate of cream-filled cannolis. A chocolate mousse cake that we'd brought down for my sister- and brother-in-law's twenty-fifth anniversary had thawed and was so shiny that I could see my face in its top glaze. My mother-in-law's apple pie was also shiny and perfect. There were raspberries in liqueur to top the cheesecake. And there was a little plastic container with fat cubes of watermelon and another of cantaloupe. I was seated in my usual place at the center of the table, surrounded by the yummiest stuff on earth. Most of the family had a little slice of everything and finished with a cannoli and a small cookie. I opted for the tiniest slice of cheesecake that was physically possible to cut and some watermelon. I felt like the most deprived person in the world. The next day, the table was set with the same desserts, with the addition of whipped cream and a bowl of fresh pineapple. See how kind they were though? That fruit was for me. And I had double portions, especially of the pineapple.

I was not so good the following Saturday, however, when I had another Thanksgiving dinner, this time with my goddess-daughter and her then fiancé. I ate turkey and a small portion of yams, green bean casserole with those crunchy, fried onion things on top, a thin sliver of sweet potato pie, and two helpings of a dessert aptly named Cherry Yum Yum—cherries, cream cheese, graham crackers. I have included this recipe for your consideration in the rear of this volume. Do not make it and keep it. Create this dish, eat a tiny portion, then donate it to a soup kitchen. Life is too short to never eat Cherry Yum Yum, but it is dangerous indeed. Very dangerous.

Being conscious about it is, I think, the key. Hallowe'en taught me a valuable lesson in personal responsibility. My friend Kayla and I have a running joke about "opening up a can of personal responsibility on your ass"—a derivation of a popular Southern saying. We both think that personal responsibility is fast becoming a lost art, and Hallowe'en was a good chance for me to test that theory for myself. One part of me wanted to embrace that sugar-lust and say—it's only once a year, surely I deserve a break from all this rigor? What could it hurt? I might have the equivalent of a hangover for a few days, but no long-term damage was probable, was it?

All that self-talking and rationalizing was very tempting. But I took the opportunity to embrace Willendorf and listen with love to my deep self. Would I have been able to binge out on sugar and then get back to the program? Probably. Would I have felt badly, both physically and emotionally? Certainly. Did I choose instead to open up a can of personal responsibility on my own ass? Yes, I did. I made a conscious choice that came out of my commitment to myself.

I won't always make good choices, but I now know that the choice really is mine. The culture is permeated with excuses for me to rationalize my way through bad choices. Maybe one day I'll need to use some of them. But not today. Not today.

Besides the sugar thing, I eat rather a lot of monounsaturated fats. I don't count fat grams, and as long as it's one of those magic monos, I don't much limit what I eat of them. I make small bowls of olive oil with garlic, and I dip a piece of toasted bread in it. No longer does canned tuna in spring water lurk on the pantry shelf. Now it's albacore in olive oil. I even borrowed my sister-in-law's grocery store card while on a visit so I could score a gallon can of cold-pressed extra-virgin olive oil.

The exception to this rule is butter. I also eat real butter on toast, on fresh vegetables, on grits. It is an indulgence, that bit of butter. And for me it has to be butter. No margarine—do you have any idea what's in that stuff? No, me neither—let's stick with natural sweet butter, shall we? There's directions for making your own butter in the section The Witch's Test Kitchen: Eats and Stuff.

I have salmon at least once a week, and I eat the aforementioned canned tuna in olive oil on a bed of spring greens. My preference in life would be to be a vegetarian, if I could grow all my own vegetables and eat them warm from the garden in season, all year long. My truth is that I limit my intake of carbohydrates and am sensible about fat, and I have to make up those extra calories somewhere. Protein. Yes, there are nonmeat ways to do that, but they mostly involve high-carbohydrate solutions. So I eat fish and poultry, a little pork and beef. I joke that I'm a chicka-fisha-tarian. My genuinely vegetarian friends don't appreciate the humor.

I honor the spirits of the animals who gave their lives so that I may live, and because I am a Pagan, after all, I also honor the lives of the vegetables that I consume. All that honoring slows down my consumption a bit and gives me time for reflective chewing, something I've found healing and quite meditative. I recommend chewing slowly, looking at your food, conversing with your companions. Eating is—or should be—a pleasure. Bite after bite of healthy nutrition, delicious fuel for your delicious machine.

Now that low-carb eating is everywhere, you have the option of buying ready-made low-carb meals and treats at your grocery store. I saw some ice cream today that has only eight grams of carbs in a half-cup serving. Look at the list of ingredients—crap, crap, crap. Better to occasionally eat a half cup of real ice cream made with nutritious cream, some sugar and vanilla than to poison your system with nonnutritive chemicals that have fewer carbs. Eat a big salad, grill a chicken breast, and then really enjoy a half-cup serving of the best ice cream you can afford.

One of my favorite treats in the long-ago, sugar-drenched glory days of my early middle age was to eat a lot of chocolate-covered cherries on Boxing Day. I was steeling myself to forsake a cherished but unhealthy tradition that first year of Willi. I managed to restrict myself to a tiny box, maybe four pieces, of handmade local chocolates, one a day for the days after Yule. That satisfied my sense of entitlement, my sense of fair trade, and my sweet tooth. Since then, I've lost the desire as well as the habit to maintain that tradition. As I write this, there is a box of chocolate-covered cherries that came as a hostess gift for a supper invitation. It has sat there, unopened, for several months while I eat fresh South Carolina peaches and Concord grapes from my backyard, fat and purple and sun warmed.

This is probably a good place to talk about portions. When you sit down to a plate of pasta, do you imagine a sea of linguini covered in rich red sauce? Does the thought of eating a half cup of pasta make you feel sad and deprived?

Yeah, me too. Thinking seriously about portions required me to keep a measuring cup handy any time I was cooking or eating. And there are some things, pasta being one, that are not at this point worth it to cook and eat. Maybe at a later date I will add pasta, albeit whole-wheat pasta, to my diet. I have to admit that I miss it. But since the portion police that ride my tail most of the time won't let me indulge in the quantity of pasta I'm accustomed to, I'd rather do without. You may find other things that trigger this same impulse in you. For one friend, it was bread. To eat a piece of toast in the morning or half a sandwich at lunchtime left her angry and forlorn. This is a woman who loves good bread, who haunted our local bakeries for rich loaves of whole grains, studded with nuts, fresh from the oven. It was simply too hard for her to have a little, and it was too hard on her body for her to have a lot. She feels it's the ultimate sacrifice, and in thinking that, she has a kind of righteous sense of humor about her "loss."

My point is that you may have things in your current diet that you will grudgingly do without even though you love them. Your friends will be awed by your willpower and supportive of your sacrifice, never understanding that it would be a greater sacrifice, to your way of thinking, to limit the portions. You are the only one who can make this decision for yourself, and I think it's a healthy decision. If you are learning to listen and trust your body, you have to honor yourself in matters like this. That you feel more deprived for limiting your intake instead of eliminating the food choice is pretty brave. Go for it, if that's what you and your deep earth self need right now.

And eating out? Ha ha ha. In order for a restaurant to survive in a very competitive business, they must give each diner an enormous quantity of food. There's a restaurant in my town that serves a "small" Greek salad that's enough food for an entire family. You can share with everyone at your table and still ask for a box to take the rest home. The amount of salad isn't such a big deal as the choice of entrée, however.

I got very good advice early on, and I happily share it here: as soon as the meal arrives, ask for a to-go box. Immediately. Nibble at your meal— and I do mean nibble—until it arrives, then divide your dinner and put half of it away. Just like that. Then you aren't tempted to graze through the whole thing. Out of sight, out of mind. And lunch for tomorrow.

Of course, the only way this works is if you make sound decisions about your entrée. Listen, always listen. What does your body want? What does the machine need today? A little more protein than usual—are you doing weight work? Or would you be best satisfied with a big salad with a chicken breast on top? Sautéed vegetables with brown rice? An omelet with Portobello mushrooms? Listen and try to override your treacherous taste buds. Or gently remind them that onions and garlic sautéed in olive oil are just as yummy as a sub on white bread.

I'm getting hungry just writing about it. But as I listen to my body, it's telling me to take a swig of cold water and remember that dinner was less than an hour ago—tofu sautéed in olive oil with a sprinkling of almonds on a bed of spinach on top of a romaine salad. Am I eating high on the hog or what?

JOURNAL NOTES

What are you eating, dear friend? And what are your intentions?

CHAPTER 7

BLISSFUL NAKEDNESS AND A LEATHER JACKET FROM GOODWILL

I am the whitest white woman that my Cherokee friend MariJo knows. Or at least that's what she claims, and my recent report from 23andMe confirms the ancestral whiteness of my family. Centuries of British ancestors in one tribe or another have produced some very fair skin. And I've never been a sun worshipper, so my stomach tends to be as white as my arms and vice versa. But a couple of years ago—with some encouragement from my outdoorsy friends—I decided to get a tan.

I haven't had a tan since one summer in college when I didn't have a job and swam during the day and played miniature golf in the late afternoon. My student ID from that fall showed a round and dark face and a curvy, sexy smile. It was a treat I thought I could, with planning and a lot of sunscreen, carefully have again, some twenty-five years later.

Carefully, carefully, the freckles connected, and I had what could optimistically be called some "color." I celebrated by buying one of those pump bottles full of oil that smells like coconut. I step out of a hot shower and spray this goo all over me and rub it in. It feels like endless summer, like drinking rum drinks in the autumn. As the level of oil goes down in the bottle, I'm adding almond oil to the pump bottle and continuing my dreams of summer. My daughter taught me how to wrap and wear a sarong, and I wore that to dinner at a Chinese restaurant. Oiled, semi-tan body wrapped in a sarong—could this be me? Oh yeah.

And I bought a leather jacket. A few weeks before I unloaded all my clothes at the Goodwill, I was checking out suit jackets at the store. I picked up three very nice ones, perfect for meetings and the rare formal occasion. Then I spied a rack with the sign Special Finds. Since my daughter was still exploring the fascinating world of slightly used shoes, I wandered over to this rack to see what was so special.

And there it was. Not biker black but a warm, slightly soiled brown. Padded shoulders, snaps. Sweet. I put down my sensible business jackets and took the leather one off its hanger. Just for fun, I tried it on. It fit, if I didn't snap it. And it smelled good and felt better. I strolled to the nearest mirror, trying to look like the kind of radically cool person who wears leather jackets.

The woman looking back at me was someone I hadn't seen before. The warm brown looked good with my brown hair. The shoulder pads were a little much but not bad. The woman in the mirror smiled, and her whole face changed. She liked the way she looked in that jacket. She liked it a lot.

So I bought it—using a credit card at the Goodwill was another first for me. And I carefully stowed it in the trunk of the car, marveling. I don't want to imply that I have a thing for leather, but my actions proved otherwise. That jacket was followed by the acquisition of a full-length black duster in Italian leather, and I am, even as we speak, scouting for a black leather jacket to replace the terribly loved and worn brown one. Biker black, this time, because I am the witch of this place and that seems somehow fitting.

It didn't stop at topcoats however. Over the course of a couple of years, I acquired three pairs of black boots and one brown for the sake of accuracy. No, silly child, no stilettos. But strapped and buckled, the last pair reaching past my knees and onto the thigh. Make of that what you will.

As your shape changes, you will find yourself with clothes that get bigger and bigger. It's magic. You start loving and listening to your body, and your body begins to change. And when you started the loving, you had a closet full of clothes that more or less fit. Later, you have a closet full of clothes that fit someone larger than you. Then the day comes when you give away most of your clothes, your closet is empty, and the choices of couture are endless.

And, to me at least, baffling.

For too many years to count, I had gone to the plus-size section of a department store and had bought something shapeless and loose-fitting. Basic pieces like pants and shirt or sweater, usually in cotton, often in black. Is that what you've been doing too? Haunting the "big and tall" or ladies department, taking things from the rack that are probably too big and not even trying them on? It's a familiar scenario for those of us who may have grown to be fashion challenged.

As you love your body into a different shape and level of fitness, you will actually find clothes that fit. Sculpted in the seat, tapered at the waist. It will be a revelation, and it may be somewhat daunting for you, as it has been for me. I finally had to admit about a month ago that I have no idea what looks good on me. I bought a couple of form-fitting blouses, and I've gotten a few pairs of pants. But beyond that, I'm not sure. I've asked a friend to go on a shopping safari with me in a month or so and help me look for my own new style.

I've also been paying attention to clothes in a way I didn't before. I notice what our customers are wearing and what my fellow shoppers at the drugstore look like. Last night, I went by the drugstore after work to get a thermometer, and the woman behind me in line looked great. A ribbed, loose turtleneck sweater and a long coat with wide-ish shoulders. Tapered and fitted slacks gave her a long, lean, and powerful look that I admired. And her hair was blown back by the wind and her cheeks flushed, adding to the look of strength and vitality.

See? I'm working this through in my head. You may be luckier than I and boldly reach for the exact right thing from the rack, but I think I'm going to need some help.

One of my healthcare providers has been helping me set some goals for myself. I don't work a lot with goals—I think of them as suggestions rather than Holy Writ—so I was unsure how to proceed when people asked—as they inevitably do—how much more are you planning to lose.

Heck, I wasn't planning to lose any. It started happening when I asked my body what she wanted, and she replied, fresh fruit. Vegetables. Water. Long walks by the river. I wasn't sure how to respond. It seemed for a while like I lost ten pounds every holy day. Pagan holidays in my tradition happen every six weeks—Solstices, Equinoxes and Cross-Quarter days. So I was losing a little more than a pound a week.

I wondered—how much should I weigh? I had a vague recollection from The President's Council on Physical Fitness in middle school (the fitness Nazis) that someone my height ought to weigh 135 pounds or so. But hadn't all that changed lately? And what the heck is a BMI? Beth, the aforementioned healthcare provider, caught me checking out the BMI chart above the sink in the exam room.

She steered me away and warned me against taking something like that to heart. Look at it this way, she began. What did you weigh ten years ago? More or less than now? More. Twenty years ago? More. Thirty years ago? I'm not sure. So, says Beth, have you ever, as an adult, weighed what you weigh now? Maybe high school, I replied. But I'm not sure. My colleague Kim assures me that I'm smaller than I was in college. Now I need to rustle up one or two of my high school chums.

We were cleaning out drawers lately and came across some clothes from my depressed-grad-student days. I tried some pants on, and they were a little big. And we found a shirt I'd worn in eighth grade that fits now.

Most amazing of all was my Baja. Remember those? Funky, hooded shirt/jackets from Mexico that every hippie in the '70s owned? Sometimes striped but mine was a solid, oatmeal color. I'd bought the largest size I could find, but it was too tight in the hips and I set it aside. It came to the light of day in the great cleanout. Well, now it fits, that Baja. And as I walk around the track at the river, I'm just another middle-aged hippie, trying to stay warm.

My daughter went through her Goth phase as I was losing the initial poundage, so I inherited the bright, colorful clothes that didn't fit her new vibe. I traded her some ultra-baggy black sweaters, and I got some T-shirts, a denim skirt, and a pair of corduroy pants to keep me warm in the winter. She offered me a couple of pairs of jeans, but they weren't quite right, as you will discover in the next chapter. I looked forward to her chucking unwanted clothes down the steps and asking me to bag them for Goodwill. I went through them first, appreciating hand-me-downs from my baby. Life does go full circle, if we can be patient and if we pay attention. Now she lives a couple of hours away, and I still manage to inherit the occasional not-quite-right garment.

I also had to have all new costumes for the madrigal group I sang with at the time, the Greenwood Consort. We had medieval costumes for the festival music, and I happily created a long princess line surcote of gorgeous brocade. I bought a chatelaine's belt to wear low on my hips, accentuating the long line at the waist. I had never been able to wear this style before because I always had too much hip and butt to pull it off. But now? It looked pretty good, if I do say so myself. We also wore formal Victorian evening wear for the winter music, and I found that I actually needed a bustle for the first time.

JOURNAL NOTES

What are you wearing and why? And what are you keeping in the back of your closet, just in case, that should rightly go to the thrift store or women's shelter?

CHAPTER 8

Few people can understand my obsession with owning a pair of Levi's. My daughter cannot disguise her disdain for my name-brand folly, but there it is. They're not the most stylish jeans, not the most economical jeans. What is it about Levi's that has me checking them out in every shop that carries them? Why is it I now know the numbers—I'm wearing 577s but aching for a pair of 501s.

I grew up poor in a world where girls wore cotton dresses or shorts and a shirt or denim overalls. I didn't start wearing jeans until high school (and for the first couple of years, girls weren't allowed to wear pants to school unless it was very cold) when I wore a size eighteen that was purchased at a local discount store called Sky City.

I remember the sales clerk was dismissive of me when I wanted a pair of blue jeans, and my choices were burgundy and purple. If she wore something smaller, she'd have more choices, she told my mother, as though I weren't there.

64

What can you expect with jeans that big? What I expect, my adult self says to that long-ago bitchy saleswoman (who probably had problems of her own and wasn't making as much money as the men who worked in the same job and maybe had a husband who wasn't worth a plugged nickel) who decided to take it out on a fat teenager who just wanted a pair of blue jeans like all the other kids had—what I expect is to be treated with a little respect and not talked to as though I'm stupid. I wasn't stupid then, and I'm not stupid now. The difference is, then I was fat and young. Now I'm slim and old enough to speak my mind. Long before I started the Willendorf program, I dropped the passive in passive-aggressive. It feels heavenly, by the way. I advise you to try standing up for yourself. It's worth the discomfort.

Now back to those Levis. Even if I could have fitted into them, such expensive jeans were out of the question on our budget, so I made do with burgundy no-name denim pants. It wasn't long before I discovered the comfort of men's jeans and switched my allegiance to the other side. I wore men's jeans for years, adjusting the too-big waist while enjoying the give in the rise. As a seamstress, I learned to make the adjustments with a minimum of bother and didn't think any more about it.

Until about forty pounds in, when I tried on a pair of loose-fitting Levi's in a generous size eighteen. They fit and were remarkably comfortable. The ratio of waist to hip was good, and I had lots of upper-thigh room.

Perfect. I bought a pair of sixteens to grow into. And then a pair of fourteens and then a pair of twelves. You want to know what I'm lusting after now? A pair of button-fly 501s. Size ten. As soon as they go on some sort of sale at my favorite department store, I'll acquire them. And at some point in the not-so-distant future, I will wear them. With a sleek little shirt that shows a little belly and a smidge of cleavage. I'll look good and feel better. And I can be compassionate toward that long-ago sales woman and that fat teenager who just wanted some jeans.

A brief coda to the Levi's story came from my sister-in-law in Atlanta. My nephew came down to breakfast one morning when we were visiting, and his mom asked him if he was still blue. He was wearing shorts and grinned a big goofy grin. We looked at his legs, and sure enough they were palest blue. Seems he hadn't washed his new Levi's before wearing them and had played a damp game of football the day before.

I figured it was like wearing woad in the olden days—a badge of a warrior's honor.

JOURNAL NOTES

What are your Levi's? What garment seems unattainable but is deeply desired?

CHAPTER 9

THE EMERGENCE OF THE BONE WOMAN—I
CAN SEE MY BONES; HOW WEIRD IS THAT?

As you might imagine, adjusting to a new body is a challenge and a delight. There's the obvious change as your clothes get looser and looser, and your friends start complaining about that big ugly shirt—thanks, Lu. I've never been a clothes horse, though I was a theatrical costume designer for most of my adult life. I can tell you who wore a farthingale and why, and I know how to drape a toga, but my personal idea of high fashion is comfortable black clothes, lots of silver jewelry, and flat shoes. I even bought a copy of *Vogue* a few weeks ago but have yet to have the courage to actually open it. Sad, really.

There came a day—and this will happen to you sooner than you know—when I gave away (or threw away, in the case of tattered, size eleven cotton underwear) all my clothes. Okay, well, most of my clothes. I kept some big ugly shirts just to spite my friends and a pair of size twenty-six jeans. But most of my wardrobe went into black garbage bags, which were ceremoniously dumped at my favorite Goodwill store. I was left with lots of exercise clothes, a couple of pairs of black pants for work, and a few work shirts.

For months I wore the same outfits over and over until I was sick of seeing them. And since I am continuing to lose weight and get fit, it seemed silly to buy clothes that I wouldn't be able to wear in two months. In fact, at Thanksgiving, my mother-in-law took me upstairs to show me some shirts she'd brought down from New York. I wasn't sure if she'd gotten them for me or herself, but as she laid them ceremoniously on the bed, I knew I wouldn't be taking them home. Though they were much smaller than anything she'd given me before, those shirts were still too big. Not right for me because of the styles and fabrics, but more importantly, they were simply too big for me. There was a time when too big was better than too small, when I'd be happy to have something that didn't bind across the hips or that could be unbuttoned and worn over a turtleneck. But those days are past, and I hugged her for thinking of me but declined the offer, I hope graciously.

In the before time, when I lost weight for whatever reason, I noticed it first in my face, where I'd acquire some cheekbones. That happened early on in this process, so early I hardly noticed it. The next thing that happened was seeing funny dents at the top of my chest. At first I only saw them in a certain light in the bathroom in the early morning. Those dents were the harbingers of my collarbones, a facet of the human body usually best viewed on those skinny little women who are soap opera stars. Their hideously inappropriate (who wears a skin-tight black cocktail frock to a business meeting?) clothes always show a maximum of collarbone and leg.

There in my own bathroom mirror on my own shrinking frame were the same collarbone dents. I watched them speculatively, as though they might reveal carved initials or traces of alien forebears. I'm feeling them right now—did you know they go out almost to the tops of your arms? No, I didn't either, but when I run my hands outward from the middle of my neck, they keep going.

I was standing behind the counter at the bookstore where I used to work when a fearsome itch started just south of my waistband in the back. Some errant polyester clothing tag was annoying my tender Irish skin. No customers being present, I slipped my hand down my back to flatten the tag.

That's when I felt a strange lump at the base of my spine. An icy chill shot through me. Lumps, as we all know, are not good. And I was at work where I could hardly ask my boss to check it out for me. And there was no way I could see it in the little mirror in the bathroom. I gingerly felt the lump again. It wasn't sore. That's good. I felt the area around it, and directly north of the first bump, I felt another. And another.

I was feeling my spine for the first time in my life. And it was pretty weird. Since then, I've discovered all sorts of bony bits in the former roundness of my anatomy. The sharpness of my hip bones never ceases to amaze me. After years of being generously padded, they are easily detectable, just by putting my hands on my hips.

One day I was sitting in the office at work with my legs crossed and my arms wrapped around my torso. One of my colleagues saw me and commented on my body language. I looked down at myself and explained that I was crossing my legs because only recently could I do that with comfort. And I had my arms wrapped around because I was exploring my rib cage. My body was not revealing my inner hostility, it was adjusting to new realities.

I first discovered the archetype of the Bone Woman in the seminal work *Women Who Run With The Wolves* by Clarissa Pinkola Estes. The Bone Woman gathers scattered bones from the desert and stores them deep in her cave. When she has found all the bones, she assembles them and selects an appropriate song with which to sing muscle and flesh onto the skeletal frame. Then she begins to sing and continues her song until the wild creature is reborn and runs free into the world. This reminds me of the creator in the Genesis story, breathing life into the red dust of the earth and bestowing freedom on living creatures.

It is up to each of us to be our own Bone Woman. As we assemble the bones—the hip bones, the cranial bones, collarbones—we must choose the appropriate song to reassemble the whole creature, wild and free.

As my feet lose the burden of hauling around all those extra pounds, I am noticing my ankles and long toes. I have thick peasant ankles and always have. But I find myself loving the sturdy elegance of these bones, as they emerge above the sides of my feet. I wiggle my long toes and appreciate the curve of my instep and my arch. I embrace this Bone Woman aspect of Willendorf as I choose the song that will breathe life and wildness into my bones again.

Being a creature of my time, I have decided to celebrate these incredible ankle bones with a tribal marking—a snake and some shamrocks for my Irish forebears. I talked it over with my friend Rebecca on the phone one cool Sunday morning. We spoke about our lives and hopes and loves, as women tend to do when having coffee on an autumn morning in leaf-peeping season. I told her about my plans for the ankle snake, and as I talked, I stroked this thick, powerful ankle of mine, my fingers tracing the shape of the snake, my fingers tapping the places where shamrocks might be. When she asked which ankle, I laughed and said, "I guess the left one. That's the one I'm drawing on with my fingers while we're talking."

You see, I'm still working the Willendorf process most every day. I keep glancing at my ankles, wondering if they'd ever "shape up," wondering if there's anything I could do to make them slim and shapely, what I described to Rebecca that morning as "Cinderella ankles." And it's not moving fast enough—though I walk and bike and massage, these thick ankles don't change much. Nor will they.

So I've decided to love and honor their glory, their power. To be enchanted by the way they work, their simple design and elegant function. Not Cinderella ankles, because these ankles would not have put up with all that crap from three people they barely knew. They practically scream get your own damn breakfast! Wash your own stinking laundry!

I've got hills to climb and rivers to swim and snakes to charm. And with my fair skin, maybe I should talk to my snake-loving biologist friend Tim and ask him to help me pick the perfect snake for these wonderful ankles. Something sinuous and colorful and totally me. He'll probably suggest a bright viper. I'll let you know how that works out.

It's autumn in the hills, and I'm cold in a way that usually doesn't happen until January. I'm sleeping alone on a couch/futon in a warm room, and I find sometimes that I can't get warm at night. My winter coat is impossible, of course. I bought it years ago, and it was big on me even then. I haven't had the guts to try it yet this year, but I know it'll be far too big and far too heavy. I had decided to do without a coat this year, to dress in layers and throw my wool cloak over the top. But these past few evenings are making me rethink that decision. I may have to check out the coats at the mall soon and see if something sings to me.

Fat people are warmer, which is a curse in the halcyon days of August but a blessing in the raw winds of February in the Appalachian Mountains. We may sweat and curse in the summer, but we make warm bed companions when the frost is on the pumpkin, as we say around here.

But now the fire in my inner furnace is dimmed. My circulation seems fine. It's the insulation that's at fault. I have an enormous pink flannel nightgown that I rarely wore in the winter. Now that I need its extra warmth, it is far too large, like getting into a thin sleeping bag and wrapping it around my frame.

What's to be done but buy something warmer? How can I dream of faraway lands and flying by night if I can't get to sleep in the cold? It's a good time to think about my ancestors in houses without central heat in a world without polar fleece. Or my long-ago ancestors living in round houses in the British Isles. They at least brought all the animals in with them, creating some creature comfort.

Maybe I should get a great hairy hound to sleep on my futon and share her warmth. What would Willendorf do? An animal pelt? A thickly woven robe, decorated with shells and gold? Her beautiful abundance is difficult to imagine enrobed, isn't it? And given her roundness, she may have been the ideal companion for her loving mate, warm as toast beneath the pelts.

We'll explore the notion of singing for a moment. You may be one of those blessed folks who simply opens your mouth and creates a beautiful sound with beautiful words to match. That, alas, cannot be said for me. So if you are, as I am, lyrically challenged, you may want to take your journal and scribble down a few verses. You may borrow verses from a poet or create your own. When you have found the right words, words that make your soul as well as your mouth sing, spend time with them, repeating them as little chants and marches as you walk or bike. Write them on a slip of paper and put them on your lovely altar space. Then use them in your meditations, spinning a tune with them if you so desire. Use them to remember that the bones are all connected, that they are covered with muscle and flesh and skin, that they house the workings of your organs. Rejoice in this framework for your sturdy earth self. Pound your heels into the dirt, wrap your arms around your frame, and feel the contours of rib and hip and pelvis. Place your cupped hands on your knees. Trace the circle of your ankles. The Bone Woman sings within each of us as we honor the song.

A life lived with the name of a famous (and infamous) romantic poet has left me reticent about writing much poetry. But here's one I did a couple of years ago. I offer it here as a way to look at the ferocity of the Bone Woman.

Bone Sister

Here She comes again.
Looking like the twisted pages of a paperback trash novel.
Yellow and sharp but still some crumbly too.
Bone Sister rides a nice car. One of those sleek and silver Lexus things
With black leather seats.

The turn signals work good
But She don't use them.
She don't like people knowing which way
She plans to head next.

Your way?
My way?
Her own way, that is for sure no lie.

Bone Sister wears a nice coat. A long black leather one.
She got it at the fine thrift store downtown.
And it fits good.
But She don't button it.
She likes to feel the sharp wind on Her ribs
And the way the sides flap behind Her
As She goes.

Your way?
My way?
Her own way, that is for sure no lie.

In the hill country,
In the hard country,
We call Her Bone Sister.
We call Her White Mamaw.
We call Her Plumb-Kilt Woman.

We call Her.
But She don't come
Til She wants to.

JOURNAL NOTES

As you approach this Bone Woman, what do you take away from the idea of bones as support, as power?

CHAPTER 10

What Do You Want: Setting Willi Goals

Me to the point—what does your body want? Remember, we're checking in with our old friend and asking the deep questions. You're doing your daily meditation, and you have learned to sit in silence. You've learned the difference between "I want Oreos and I want them right now!" and "Gosh, when I eat an apple every morning, I make it through to lunch with energy and a clear mind. Maybe I'll make this a regular part of my nutritious breakfast!"

Because every body is different. Okay, some bodies are remarkably similar—you and your best friend may both have good results by swimming and adding more protein to your diet. But even you and your best friend have different bodies—different metabolisms, different food preferences, different exercise programs that you can stick with.

As you will remember from previous chapters, my initial goals—my Willi goals—were to lower and stabilize my blood sugar without medication.

This required a diet transformation and a course of regular, though not terribly strenuous, activity.

When that Willi goal was achieved—and blessedly seems to be holding—my body was already on the weight-loss train. So it seemed only sensible to think in terms of setting some weight loss and some general fitness goals.

As I embraced Willendorf, I also embraced forty years of often conflicting diet information. A nutritionist helped me with the latest thought of what to eat and what not to eat, giving me the priceless advice about eating smaller portions. But there was still a lot of confused ninth grade health class information about how much someone my height "should" weigh, what kind of exercise achieves results, and whether or not I could do this without my vicious PE teacher shaming me in front of all my friends.

I didn't set particular weight-loss goals but clothing-size goals. I wanted to end up wearing a size ten dress pants and size twelve jeans. But here I am, suspecting I'm going to lose at least ten more pounds, and I've already achieved those goals. So instead of concentrating on size, now I'm concentrating on getting some muscle. I'm learning where deltoids and triceps are through boring and painful repetitions with a dumbbell. I've decided "six-pack abs" aren't quite me, but I do crunches every other day to tighten up my abdomen for those hip-hugging Levis I love.

It has helped me immeasurably to keep a record of the exercises I try and what seems to be working and what I can't and won't do. My little Willendorf journal shows me the highs and lows (as well as the painful encounters) of my road to fitness. I've created some exercises because they felt good when I moved that way only to later discover that the movement has a name and is regularly used by all sorts of people to do the very thing I want done. It's just another case of being willing to take a chance and trust my body. I can't stress enough that this always works. You really do know what you need to know. But you may not know that you know it!

Take up your journal now and consider what your goals could be. Take a break from all this reading and spend some time with your fine self. Do some coloring or singing or dancing. Then come back to this Willi business refreshed.

JOURNAL NOTES

CHAPTER 11

HITTING THE WALL

There came a point where everyone was saying "You've lost more weight! Wow!" yet I hadn't lost an ounce. I spent an entire month losing, gaining and re-losing the same four pounds. Up I'd go, down I'd go. No matter what I ate or didn't eat. No matter how much I exercised or didn't exercise. The same four pounds.

I had the optimistic fantasy that by working out, I was rearranging fat and adding muscle, which, as all fat people know, weighs more than fat. Wasn't that some sort of muscle there on the side of my leg? Wasn't that pendulous flesh under my upper arms slightly less pendulous than it used to be? Hmmm. I could fool myself into thinking I was firming up, but the scale didn't lie. Those four pounds were stopping me in my tracks.

I had hit the wall. And let me tell you, it sucked.

I tried fewer calories and more exercise. My weight actually went up. I was told that for the amount of exercise I was getting, I needed to up my caloric intake. Wait a minute—you as my doctor are telling me to eat more? How can this be possible? She laughed at me, as she often does.

Try it. See what happens. I did. I ate two hundred additional calories that day, and the next day I noticed a slight change in weight. Within a week, I'd lost a couple of pounds.

Now I'm yo-yoing again. I'm down from where I was before, but the yo-yo continues. I have to come to terms with the fact that what was once steady and relatively easy is now less regular and harder. Since my goal was not specific amounts of weight loss, it is not traumatic so much as annoying.

But I decided to practice what I've been preaching and listen to my body. I went down to my favorite river park and took a walk, ending at a wooden overlook with a little bench. I leaned over the railing and stared at the river, and I asked my body what was up. No, I didn't do it aloud. I took some deep breaths, spoke the Cherokee name of the river, and listened.

I heard crows, and I heard wind in the trees. And what I heard from my body, from my deep earth self, was this: cut me some slack, for pity's sake! I'm working overtime here, processing wholesome food, converting that food to energy, hauling us around this track and into the woods and out to play pool, wherever we want to go and play. I am adjusting to all this, and it takes some time. So give me some time. Keep doing what you're doing, and I'll keep doing what I'm doing, and we'll be fine. Calm down, woman. This is life, not the Boston Marathon. Enjoy! Did we bring the water bottle?

See how wise my body is?

I am evidently a slow learner because I had to learn this lesson again, in the first real snowfall of the season the first year of Willendorf. My daughter woke early, gleeful about missing school and having time to recheck her social studies project (which, of course, she did not do because she spent the day off playing in the snow, hanging out with her friend Erika, watching DVDs).

I check my weight every day. At this time, I was in one of those plateau periods where I had gained and lost the same few pounds over and over and had come to the conclusion that I looked fabulous, felt fabulous and was, in general, fabulous. And, moreover, if I could get through the eat-a-thon of Yuletide in Appalachia without actually gaining weight, I'd be ahead of the game. So no worries.

Let this next confession serve as a warning. Remember I was still early on in this process and still working at the bookstore, though that is hardly a good excuse. I had gotten my work schedule for the holidays—different days off, some longer hours, the annual store birthday party—and also began planning our circle's seasonal celebration for the solstice. At the same time, I and my business partners were planning a pilgrimage to Britain scheduled for the following spring. So yes, there was unusual pressure. But nothing compared to what I was about to put myself through.

The world was silent and still. I had a day ahead of me at home to do some holiday preparations. I ate half a banana, went to the bathroom for my workout clothes and, while naked, stepped on the scale.

I had gained two pounds.

And I freaked out.

I immediately planned to double my exercise for the day, to starve myself into submission. All I could see in the day before me were endless opportunities to eat. I could see myself getting larger and larger until I had to go back to Goodwill and buy back all my old clothes. I saw myself sick and pathetic and…

This is the result of hubris. Do you know about hubris? It was familiar to me from classical Greek dramas, all of which had characters who suffered from this problem. It is the pride that goes before a fall. It is that cocky feeling that we in the South call "the Big Head." It's the arrogant sense of superiority that always gets you in the worst trouble.

You see, I thought I was immune to those things that happen to most dieters—weight creep, lack of confidence, sabotaging friends. I was the exception, and everyone said so. I was the amazing Byron, the poster child for taking control of your life and health, the zealot of listening to your body's needs and loving yourself exactly as you are.

This could not be happening to me.

I had fallen victim to my own hype, and here I was, on the scale, regaining all the weight I had lost. There was no way out of it: I was going to have to punish myself and get my willful body into submission.

I dragged myself to the exercise bike because my usual walk was out of the question in the snow. Water bottle in hand, I planned a long, lonely bike ride, beating myself up along the way.

And then a funny thing happened, and I can't tell you how often this is the case. As I exercised, I felt better. I felt stronger and less freaked out. Then I felt happy. Ah, endorphins. Beautiful, spontaneous endorphins.

My body was doing its exercising thing, and my mind was calming down, and I was starting to judge the "situation" without fear. I looked out the window and saw the snow. We had been blessed with a remarkably warm autumn, and it had only recently gotten cold in the mountains.

Pedal, pedal, pedal. The weather was supposed to clear up later in the day, but it would still be chilly.

It hit me at about mile two. I had been thinking the day before that my metabolism didn't seem to be set on "hummingbird" lately. I didn't get ravenously hungry right before mealtimes or need to carry an apple with me at all times to fuel the machine.

Winter. Cold. Metabolism. As a woman who carefully follows the cycle of the seasons, I was being awfully dim. My body knew though, and as I pedaled, I asked myself about this hypothesis that was forming.

You reckon we're slowing down for the winter? Not hibernation per se, but conserving all that precious energy because we need to stay warm in this new season?

Yep, I reckon, came the response.

I had berated myself and terrified myself and been meaner to myself than I had during this whole process. I had rushed to judgment and condemnation because of two pounds, the very thing I've been telling people I wasn't doing. I felt a little guilty and a little ashamed. And then I finished my biking, drank a bunch of water, and started the day again. With love and trust, the Wiccan way.

There will be times when this happens in my life and in your life. We will react out of fear, and it won't be pretty. We'll lose our sense of humor and take ourselves far too seriously. I hope you will have the presence of mind to remember what you've been doing and not run screaming through the house, clutching a water bottle. But if it takes you a while to remember, you're not alone. Don't forget to breathe. Don't forget to listen. And try not to freak out.

And I will try to practice what I preach.

So I keep on doing what I'm doing, and I give myself the luxury of time. I'm not on some frantic schedule to fit into a size eight dress for the prom. I'm changing my whole life. I'm embracing the sweetness of doing and playing and living. I got all the time in the world.

So do you.

Coda: Sugar Bliss, the Acceptable Addiction

In researching this chapter, I kept asking myself and others if sugar is, technically speaking, an addictive substance. Certainly I find it to be. After all this time, I still haven't managed to totally cut it out of my diet. I still occasionally have a square of dark chocolate or a helping of Cherry Yum Yum.

In recent years, there was a study done at Rockefeller University that is quoted on a website called Sugar Shock. This study seems to indicate that sugar is indeed addictive and that ingesting it forces your body to rob needed nutrients from your bones and organs in order to process the poison you just took in the form of chocolate cake.

The websites I visited all took this very seriously and made many accusations about the sugar industry and the abuse of this delicious white substance. I learned something of the history of refined white sugar, and let me tell you, it's not a pretty sight. The more I learned about sugar, the more I understood how dreadful it is for our bodies, for the body politic, and for the environment.

But it is very, very yummy. That's the problem. Candy, cake, pie, soda, breakfast cereals, soft drinks. And that doesn't begin to touch on all the processed food products that are loaded with "hidden" sugar. Things you'd never suspect, like sugar snap peas. I'm a gardener, and every spring sees me happily planting row after row of sweet peas. They are brought in the house and steamed or sautéed or served fresh in salads. I never in my wildest dreams ever considered adding sugar to peas. What kind of sick world do we live in when tender sweet peas aren't sweet enough? In the weird world of frozen food—you know, that place where you buy peas out of season?—sugar is added to sugar snap peas. To make them sweeter.

I'm not pretending to be an expert on sugar or its effects on human physiology. I'm not even sure if it is addictive for the average person. What I do know is the affect that sugar has on me. You'll note I use the present tense, not the past one. Though I don't use sugar regularly or often, I have been unable, after all this time working the Willendorf program, to totally eradicate it from my diet. It is something I really want to do, but for now I am content that my use of refined sugar is at least limited.

Here is the problem for me, the thing that sends warning bells sounding in my head every time I indulge in sugar and why I know that, for me, it is an addictive substance. I can go weeks without sugar and not want it. Then I'll consciously decide to have an ounce of dark chocolate or a skinny slice of cake at someone's birthday. There isn't a spike in blood sugar; there isn't a weight gain. But the next day I want some more. I tell myself it didn't hurt me on Sunday, so why don't I have some more?

And that little voice scares me because I know what a toxic substance I'm considering ingesting. I worry that one day my positive self-talk won't talk me out of having a sugary dessert the next day or honey in my porridge. And I know it could all end with my driving down the road with a bag of miniature candy bars on the seat beside me, powering up with empty and dangerous calories that will only wreck my health and make me miserable.

That sounds like addict-talk to me.

JOURNAL NOTES

What food or foods create cravings for you? Are you able to avoid them or at least minimize them?

CHAPTER 12

THE NATURE OF SPELLWORKING—GOOD HEALTH, LEAN MUSCLE MASS, AND FIVE MORE POUNDS

Harry Potter is botha blessing and a curse for people like me. I get phone calls, texts and e-mails from people all the time wanting me to teach them a love spell or do an exorcism on their trailer. I am not kidding about that. I got a phone call a couple of years ago from someone who had heard I was "real good" and wanted to tell me about the weird noises and goings-on in her double-wide. I did go out and do some energy clearing, but she was expecting the kind of fireworks that real Witches don't produce. I expect she was disappointed that I didn't arrive by broomstick, wearing a pointy hat and carrying a Mason jar of goat's blood.

I got a call last year from a disgruntled woman who wanted me to kill her lawyer. With magic. She wanted me to whip up some big bad juju and get rid of this guy who was not doing his best work for her case. I spent a long time talking to her about ethics and personal responsibility and suggested that if she had problems with this guy, she should call her local bar association or at least the Better Business Bureau. She did not hear a single word I said but responded with, "Well, if you won't do it, can you teach me how to?"

Our notions about how magic works are informed by things as wide-ranging as *The Wizard of Oz* and the six o'clock news. Movies like *Charmed*, *The Craft*, and *The Blair Witch Project* (don't get me started) add fuel to the fire and confusion to the general compost of the situation.

This is not a book about the uses of magic. But I do successfully utilize energy work in the Willendorf process, so I want to introduce you to some helpful techniques for energy working. Magic—or at least the brand that I practice—is the focus of your will into energy that is used with a specific intention or set of intentions. In one aspect, it's similar to the familiar Western concept of prayer. You establish within yourself what your needs are, you give thanks for the bounty given, and you beseech your particular Deity for help in acquiring what you need, whether it's healing for someone you love or a new job or peace of mind. You might repeat that prayer for a prescribed amount of time, or it might be a one-time-only need.

My field is folk magic, specifically Appalachian folk magic, the subject of my first two books. It is filled with simple and practical magic techniques that always begin with setting a firm intention. That's how magic works. You determine your goal. You reach into and around yourself to tap into the energy that is all around us all the time. Then you project your will by using that energy to achieve the results you intend.

There are many techniques for tapping into the energy, and as you practice them, you'll find that it gets easier to tap in and that there comes a time when the techniques can be simplified and still be very effective. The first step—as in all things—is to come to a quiet place in yourself through breathing and meditation.

Not breathing again. That breathing stuff is getting on my nerves. Why does everything start with breathing? Well, because everything does. Breathing connects us instantly, not only with ourselves but with the world around us, as we literally take part of that "outside" world into our lungs, giving us, it is to be hoped, vital gases to run the machine. So when the automatic process is done in a conscious way, we begin to give ourselves a powerful, grounded, and quiet place in which to live in the world in a meaningful way.

Does that help?

Okay, start with breathing. Deep, slow breathing. The kind of breathing where your belly rises and falls as your lungs fill with air all the way to their bottoms. As your lungs fill and your body feels confident that it has the necessary gas to run your engines, you'll start to relax.

Amazing, isn't it? Most people take rapid and shallow breaths so that our bodies are in a constant state of stress wondering if the next breath will be sufficient unto the day. How crazy is that? In a world where the guy driving the car in front of yours is talking on his cell phone while eating a candy bar and weaving in and out of traffic or where you bounced a check because you are math challenged or where your teenager's favorite new expression is "I hate you"—in this stressed-out world, we actually give our bodies a dose of extra stress by not breathing efficiently.

You breathe, you relax, you connect with your deep earth self, the same space you go when you embrace Willendorf and find the courage to love yourself. That connection spirals out from you into the world that supports and sustains you. You begin to tap into the energy that flows around us all the time.

Now you must be clear in your intent. No, it's not *The Monkey's Paw*—you can't phrase it the wrong way and do magical damage to yourself. But you're working to be as efficient as possible— in what you eat and how you exercise—so let's utilize some of this efficiency by being clear with ourselves about what we want.

I have used a little chant as I walk around the park. I say it to myself, usually when beginning a new lap—good health, lean muscle mass, and five more pounds. Repeat, repeat. I keep repeating it to myself until my body starts to march as I walk, like a recruit with a lively drill instructor or a tuba player in the high school marching band. Good health, lean muscle mass, and five more pounds.

For a while I was very specific about the number of pounds. If I weighed 192 and wanted to get below 190, I'd say "good health, lean muscle mass, and three more pounds." But as I was going through my rapid weight-loss phase, this was hard to keep up with. And when I hit the wall, it got to be depressing... and four more pounds. No wait, five more pounds. No, only two.

Blech. So I stick with five, figuring that's a nice round number and easy to remember. I'm looking forward to changing the chant to "good health, lean muscle mass." That will come, I think, in the distant but obtainable future.

Practical magic. As a garden-variety Witch, I appreciate the use of simple magics like this. Other simple magics you can employ as you work with Willi are self-blessings when you shower and gratitude for and blessings of your food.

You are loving yourself, aren't you? So when you peel out of your jammies in the morning and leap into a hot shower, do you take a moment to look in the mirror and acknowledge your work and love your body? I hope so. I've been doing this funny dance of looking at my shrinking butt, jiggling my wobbly underarms, poking my collarbones, and smiling at my silliness. Your next step is to feel the flow of that marvelous water as you step into the shower and honor that element. Take a second to think: water is good. As you shampoo your hair, put your hand on top of your head and bless yourself. Yep, bless yourself. Say something simple like "blessings" or something sweet like "bless-a-baby" (my mom used to say that sometimes) or a long poem like "Here I stand, as the water of life flows over me, blessing me with the element of the west. I stand firmly on the earth, I breathe the warm rich air, my water is heated by the fire of the south. In all ways, on all days, I am blessed and grateful."

Yeah, maybe that's a bit much. I might choose to do that on a day when I had a little more time or had some scary or impossible thing to do or when I was feeling a little low and sad. But do try a shower blessing—it can set the tone for your whole day or help you have good dreams.

Food is fuel for the marvelous machine—wholesome calories that keep you moving and loving and experiencing your great life. My attitude toward food changes with each passing day. Sometimes I only eat because my belly is growling and I have to. Sometimes I eat because the juiciness of a mango must be devoured in the dappled sunshine of a mountain trail. Sometimes I complain—as I did this morning while walking in the park—that none of the food I eat tastes good anymore. And sometimes I plot and scheme about how I can create the perfect loaf of bread or a cheesecake with goat cheese.

Food, as we've said before, is important. And as you switch from empty calories to whole foods, acknowledge that transition with a blessing of your food. When my daughter was a baby, she would throw her arms into the air and invoke the specific Deity with a shout "Pizza gods! Green bean gods!" Her polytheistic food universe was peopled with helpful beings who always supplied the yummiest stuff imaginable. Her happy face was prayer enough, but her enthusiasm was absolutely contagious. Now that she's a young adult, I'm not sure about her Deity choices, but I hope she still finds the food world an exciting place filled with loving and helpful friends.

Now maybe you silently repeat that childhood prayer as you pick up your fork—"God is great, God is good. Let us thank him for our food. By his hands we all are fed. Give us, Lord, our daily bread. Amen." Even as a non-Christian, I feel the love and honor present in this little chant. Anything that's been repeated as often as this has to have a lot of power. So continue that, if it is your way of honoring the Infinite with gratitude in your heart. There are also books of simple graces that can be said over your meal. My personal preference is to hold my hand over the bowl or plate or hold the mango aloft and think for a moment of the life-giving sun and water and soil that gave it form. To say thanks for the gift and the sacrifice of the giver. To remember those who grew, picked, and shipped the food, if it doesn't come from my own backyard.

So that's your crash course in the uses of magic and some simple techniques that I and others have used in a variety of circumstances when faced with diverse needs. It is nothing to fear, but it also won't make you into a Hogwarts graduate. You won't be able to amaze your guests with a swish of a magic wand. But you will be able to keep your focus on the intentional health of the body you call home.

That, for me at least, is some big juju.

JOURNAL NOTES

This might be a good place write a prayer or intention for mealtimes. Or two or three.

CHAPTER 13

There is a remarkably beautiful place in western North Carolina. Actually, there are thousands of remarkably beautiful places in my home country. But the place I'm talking about here is a large stand of old-growth forest called the Joyce Kilmer Memorial Forest. It's in the western part of the state in Swain county. This forest was set aside in 1936 after the chief of the forest service described it as one of the "very few remaining tracts of virgin hardwood in the Appalachians." And recommended "we ought to buy it to preserve some of the finest original growth in the Appalachians." So the government did, and we now have this large stand of old trees to enjoy.

The forest is named, of course, for the poet who wrote "I think that I shall never see/A poem lovely as a tree." He died in Europe in the First World War. Kilmer is full of oaks, yellow poplars, big hemlocks, and maples. There are dying giants all over the place, and the pamphlet you pick up in the parking area warns hikers against going in to the forest on windy days or after ice storms. Good idea since the limbs on those trees are bigger than a lot of the trees most of us know.

We used to go there in college sometimes. It's a long drive from Asheville, and we were always up for a road trip to the big woods. There's not much "civilization" there—just funky old trails and amazing old trees. My daughter and a friend and I took an excursion out to Kilmer the summer after I started this Willendorf program. I felt the need to get out among creatures older and bigger than myself, to walk steep trails and put my feet in cold creeks. I needed a dose of nature to get myself reconnected.

There's a strange thing that happens when you dramatically change the physical body you've been living in for many years. You start to feel a harsh disconnect, not only with yourself but with your past and with the things around you. You look in the mirror and see someone looking back at you that is not entirely familiar to you but is also not a stranger. You examine parts of your body that look different. You see things you haven't seen in years or maybe ever before.

That makes sense, doesn't it? But you also find yourself dealing with the alien experience of lean muscle mass, an altered center of gravity, and the wonder of moving backward in time.

You've lost, say, twenty pounds, and you now weigh what you weighed right after your child was born. You may find yourself thinking about that time, talking to friends about it, reliving it.

You may begin to think of yourself as the age you were when you weighed that amount. You will find yourself "youthening" as the process continues.

I hope you will find new ways to celebrate how you are now and will remember with gentleness and, if necessary, some humor, the person you were then. You may find yourself wistful for days gone by, and this may be a time for you to recapture some of those old rowdy feelings. To remember yourself a little nearer to wholeness through the youthening process. Enjoy, my dear.

Let me try to explain. Your *self*, in my opinion, is the muscle and bone and guts of you, as well as the spirit that resides within and around you. So when you dramatically change your physical self, there must be changes in the spiritual self as well. My friend DeerEyes, who practices a traditional Cherokee spirituality, says that the change really occurs on the inside first and then is mirrored in the physical plane. Not being a Cherokee shaman, I don't know if this is how it always worked. But I do know that when I heard the results of my blood work on the phone, I didn't get scared or go into denial. My entire life simply… changed. When people comment on my successful weight loss and fitness program, they sometimes say, "It must have been very hard." But it wasn't hard, not the way they are imagining.

Don't think I've got some sort of monstrous willpower or force of character that got me through this immensely hard thing. I knew my life had to change, and so I changed it. Yes, breaking my sugar addiction was hard. But as you learned in the Introduction to this book, I somehow intuited that I could replace the craving for sugar with a plunge into dried whole fruits. I didn't do a Google search or research it in a medical library. I knew instinctively what my body needed to make this cellular-level change. And I gave it to myself. And you may be doing the same thing.

Good for you, by the way.

Let me return with you to the big woods. We had heard the double loop trail at Kilmer described as a "granny trail." That must have been one hell of a granny because the combination of heat and humidity made it challenging for all three of us. We swatted bugs and looked longingly at the little wild creek that plunged through the base of the hill below the trail. At one point, I gave in to my willful younger self and scampered off the path, down the hill, and into the creek. It was worth the uphill hike back to the trail. The water was cold and fragrant and reviving.

The trees are magnificent. No, they're not California redwoods, but they are taller and wider and older than most other trees I've seen. I confess to several bouts of tree hugging and one period of sitting beneath this enormous old poplar and leaning my tired back against its trunk. There was a gnarly frog near me in the dense bark, and I watched her, almost completely camouflaged in the bark and perfectly still. I wondered how it must be to live in that body, with its strong haunches and bulging eyes. And I also wondered if the frog made a conscious decision to be still in my dangerous human presence or if it was instinct. I stretched my legs and left both tree and toad behind. Sitting is not as comfortable as it once was—there's less sit-upon on my posterior to sit upon.

Not only do you have all this adjusting to do, you have friends and family who aren't quite sure what to make of the whole thing. Some will be quietly doubtful, some will be more blatant.

Most people don't like change. We fear it because we feel out of control and because we can't be sure of the ultimate outcome. We fear change because, in the words of the Bard of Avon, we "would rather bear the ills we have, than fly to others we know not of." So there may be people in your life who miss the "old" you, and I am being charitable about that.

There's someone I know who pushes a lot of buttons for me. She has been a friend and a business partner and a circle sister, and she drives me crazy most of the time. She loves one-upmanship. If I say I have a degree in paleontology, then she has two and is a guest lecturer at the Museum of Natural History. If I spent a week in London, she lived there for a month and no one ever suspected she was an American. You get the picture—someone whose self-esteem is so low she must compensate constantly, must compete even with the people she loves so that she's always on top.

One of my Willi goals was to squirm my sumptuous hips into size fourteen pants. So when I reached that, I told my nearest and dearest, expecting them to celebrate my victory. Almost everyone did—except One Up. Her response was—fourteen? I can't believe it. I'm a twelve, and you're much bigger than me. You can't be a fourteen.

Now, to be fair, she wasn't doubting my word. She was coming face-to-face with the reality that the woman she had always thought of as "fatter than me" really wasn't anymore. Some of your friends, acquaintances, and family—what I like to refer to as "kith and kin"—will feel threatened by the changes in your body. They'll feel that way for a variety of reasons—your new body may make them feel inadequate because they haven't achieved the same thing, or they may have always had you as the benchmark of "as long as I'm not as fat as X, I'm not really that fat." My mother would've said they were jealous, but I think it's even deeper than that.

You changing your life may mean that you will put up with less crap from them. It may mean that you'll have such deliciously powerful self-esteem that they can't hurt you to feel better about themselves. There are all sorts of reasons that people will want you to not change.

Some of them will try to sabotage what you're doing with clever quips or offers of food. Others will openly criticize where you've gotten in your program. They are the ones who will remind you that you still have those saddlebags and that they are very difficult to get rid of. Or they will caution you about eating too many apples, because even though they are very good for you, they still have calories.

If your experience is similar to mine, there will be people in your life who take a sudden interest in you because you are thinner. Those people may have been lukewarm toward you when you were fat and happy. They may have ignored you in spite of your best and bubbliest personality traits. Some of those people in my life were folks I'd written off months or years ago, figuring they didn't like me for whatever reason. I'd get philosophical and think—not everyone has to like me, it's no big deal. It's not a reflection on me—it's a chemistry thing.

But it turns out it was a reflection on me. There were some people who didn't want to associate with me, couldn't even be friendly toward me because I was fat. This has been a horrific revelation to me, honestly it has. And my shock has been borne out in discussion with one of my circle sisters, Terri. She and I are shrinking together, giggling about sizes, and smirking about how tough and disciplined we've become. "No," says she. "I can't stay to chat. I've got to get to the Y." And we both laugh like maniacs, cackle like Witches.

We weren't cackling, however, when she shared that a coworker had gotten awfully chummy since her weight loss began. I can't remember if this coworker actually said she liked her better now that she isn't so fat, but this person certainly gave Terri that impression. Can you imagine not liking someone because they're fat? Maybe you can. I can't. I dislike people who are mean or shallow or condescending, but I don't recall ever disliking someone because of their weight. Skinny people—I'm fine with them. Tall people—they're okay. You already know I like round bodies. Maybe it's my Pisces sun sign, but I don't get it. Maybe I never will.

I am blessed with an incredible support network of friends, family, and acquaintances. With few exceptions, they have cheered me on every step of the way and listened to me as I talked on and on about the Willendorf program. They call me "skinny" and proclaim my youthful appearance throughout the land. When I use one of my favorite retorts—they can kiss my wide, white, Irish, Pagan, Appalachian ass—most people will giggle a bit, and some will say it's not so wide, you know. Not anymore.

Surround yourself with a big team of cheerleaders, and get rid of or ignore the people who want you to fail for their own agenda. Either excuse yourself from their lives or shut them up with charm or—as every grandmother advises—just ignore them.

Too bad for them that this is your body and your decision. Keep listening to your heart, and smile graciously at the vicious little snipes. Living well really is the best revenge. And now that I wear a size twelve and am moving toward a—gasp!—ten, my friend seems a little less harsh. I think she's getting used to the change. So another lesson is—be as patient with the people around you as you are with yourself.

Unless they push one button too many.

Then you may need a long hike in the big woods. Put your trusty water bottle in your day pack, throw in a mango and some crackers, and head for the hills. There's nothing like a splash in the creek, a breathless uphill walk on a granny trail to get your whole little self into some sort of perspective. Trees are loving and gentle companions who don't mind the occasional hug. Or you can try your own variation on the invitation to kiss your hind end.

JOURNAL NOTES

Where is your power place? Where do you go to feel connected to the wide world? Where do you feel safe?

CHAPTER 14

TEST DRIVING THE MASERATI—DID I JUST CRACK A RIB?

This, my friends, is a cautionary tale. Proceed with care.

One of the pleasures of listening to your body, stabilizing your weight and getting fitter, is that you are rewarded with buckets of energy. When you give your body less bulk to carry around and when you give it more muscles to do its work, you'll experience surges of quite remarkable energy. You may stay up later and go out into the world more often (whether hiking or shopping or simply walking about). There may even come a time when you have so much energy that you'll be tapping your foot, just to have something to expend it on.

This is when you know that your late model, usually reliable sedan has turned into a Maserati. And you'll naturally want to take it out on the open road and see what it can do. You'll be taking your morning walk along the river and you'll break into a run, just to see if you can without falling over. You'll eye the maple tree at the back of the driveway and wonder how far up it you can climb.

I have known Connie and David for years. They are good friends of my oldest friend Michael, and I love them both. They have a daughter named Maranda, who I have seen grow from a scrappy little girl to a feisty young woman. Her son, Jamie, was entering the same elementary school that my daughter was leaving, so we reconnected as parents and served on a couple of committees together. She's a great storyteller—a traditional Appalachian skill that comes very naturally to Maranda. After committee meetings, she'd tell funny stories about her women's rugby team.

I've never been an athlete. In fact, jocks weren't something I even thought of as human when I was an artsy/intellectual nerd in high school. So I didn't know much about rugby—"rugby players eat their dead" is a bumper sticker I saw once, which may be the extent of my rugby knowledge. Oh, and rugby shirts.

But she made it sound like so much fun that when I saw her after losing fifty or so pounds, I asked if I could come watch one of their matches with an eye to playing. Sometime. The darling girl smiled, looked at me sadly, and shook her head.

You can watch anytime—I'd love to have you there. But Byron, you're too, um, old for rugby. It's rough—we get hurt all the time. Bloody noses, broken bones, sprains.

I was crushed. Look at this fit and muscular body, I wanted to cry out. It's just cruising for a bruising. I'm tough. I can take it. But Maranda's right. After years of sneering at jocks, one can hardly begin the process of jockdom with a sport as cheerfully brutal as rugby. So it was a short-lived dream that I ruefully share. This year I was thrilled however to attend rugby practice with Maranda and her coach husband Gary and watch their young sons being cheerfully brutal. Tradition is important, as you know.

In the quest to work my upper body as much as I do my lower, I'm constantly on the lookout for upper arm exercise. I was standing in my solarium one day, thinking about who knows what, when I spotted my daughter's bow on top of the wardrobe. Let me backtrack a bit. My daughter has a friend who loves archery, and so she wanted to try it. For her birthday last year, I bought her a young adult compound bow, which is the style of bow her friend shoots. Kate could barely draw it and soon grew tired of Robin Hood fantasies, given the size and number of mosquitoes in our back yard. So the bow and quiver are stored on the top of the wardrobe.

I thought about that bow. I thought what good upper-arm exercise archery must be. I used to do some target practice in my misspent youth and had a pretty good eye. So I gleefully took down the bow, straightened my forearm, got my left breast out of the way, and drew it back.

It was hard. A compound bow is difficult to draw at first, and then the pulleys and gears kick in and the last part is smooth and easy.

Deceptively easy. I did what you should never ever do. I turned the string loose, without an arrow in it. I was inside—I couldn't shoot an arrow in the solarium!

The bow had a kick like a mule. Like the shotgun I learned to shoot as a kid. My whole arm went boing. It was great! So I took down the quiver and went outside this time to the yard. I dropped the quiver to the ground, pulled out an arrow, aimed at the toolshed-cum-chicken house, and fired.

Whack! I was juiced. Another arrow. I felt the muscles flexing in my soon-to-be-powerful arms. I aimed again and let loose the arrow. I stood in the dappled shadows of Sherwood Forest, and the world was green and good.

As we all know, the third time's the charm. I picked up another arrow, fitted it to the bow, and pulled. I felt a tearing all along my rib cage on the right side. Holy moly. I let the arrow fly—and did not hit the tool shed—and gripped my torso. I wasn't at all sure what I'd done, but it really, really hurt. Like I'd cracked a rib. And to add insult to injury, I had to go retrieve those three arrows that seemed now so far away. When you become more active, someone told me later, there's always the chance that you might hurt yourself. She said this with a straight face, but I know she laughed when I left the room.

116 · H. BYRON BALLARD

JOURNAL NOTES

Finding some sort of physical activity that you enjoy, that you look forward to doing, goes a long way toward your loving, healthy goals. What are yours?

CHAPTER 15

Do I Have to Uncoil My Kundalini? Where is it Anyway?

Rituals
All acts of love and pleasure
All acts of love and pleasure
All acts of love and pleasure
These are my rituals!

In black though clad, I shone like the Moon.
At the dark end of yesterday, I shone like the Moon.
Bright.
As I glowed, as I shone, as I danced through the rain and onto the great porch of the Temple,
I was singing.
I sung a song of the coming night, long awaited.
He rose to meet me.
He rose from his place in the shadow to meet me.

The boy who was rose to meet me
And we embraced on the porch of the Temple.
The boy put his hand in mine.

"We are here again. Together as before, long time before. I have the evening free, and you have only to go home to your mother."
My thoughts ranged to the night—free me of the serpent, wild bull, free me. Stay away from field and house and play with me.

"You shine in beauty, you glow as the Moon glows in the hills. I am only in shadow, waiting, always waiting.
Tonight my waiting has been broken with the delight of you."

We will watch the cooling rain from here, but our passion will not be cooled.
The touch of finger on face, of lip to nipple, all will be enjoyed.
You must have a place, a quiet place where noise of flesh to flesh may joyfully be made.
In this place I will make for you a beautiful bed, soft with herbs from the mountains.
There we may play the lapis flute, the bowl of amber. There the animal calls and the bird calls.
There may the calls of our wild kindred be made by the priestess and the boy.

This is my praise-song through the Great Priestess. This is my praise-song promised in exchange for rain.

I have closed the gate behind me.

The garden is secured from animals and the
beans and melons are there to pick and enjoy.
I have closed the gate behind me and I walk with
a light step, a joyful dancing girl-step.
His work it is to bring the sacred oil,
To drop it slowly on the ground of honor.
Cypress oil, and dragon's blood.
Wine from grapes is his and flesh of boar.
Dumuzzi!
Whose song is joy and bliss,
Whose home smells of good things and of honey.
The boy who was remembers the way to heaven.
He remembers the words of bliss.
Dumuzzi!
Lay your head upon my breast.
Sweet is the growth of the vine, permission given.
The taste of thin broth fills my mouth as the night
cools to morning.

This is my praise-song through the Great
Priestess. This is my praise-song promised in
exchange for rain.
            —*From the pen of your author and occasional poet*

Okay, this is the chapter on sexy underwear
and orgasm. You may either skip it or read it
first. Whatever works for you.

I was invited to be a speaker at a ladies'
luncheon. Given my rough beginnings as a child
without an indoor bathroom, this was kind of
sweet to me. I was invited to this lovely private
home in an exclusive enclave on top of a mountain

to be an "expert voice" in the field of ancient and modern Goddess worship, something I speak and write about with some frequency.

I chose my clothes carefully, as working-class people tend to do in the presence of the gentry. I avoided my patented black clothes and silver jewelry shtick and instead chose something flowing and artsy. Simple, elegant jewelry. I was ready for the mountain.

I had given up trying to wear my old and very large underwear and had bought a few pairs of lacy little things that passed for undergarments at that store in the mall with angel wings in the window. I guessed at the size—I used to be an eleven so was I now an eight? A six? I bought the six, assuming that if it didn't work, it would soon. When I tried it on at home, it seemed to cover all the bits and bobs, so I put it in my drawer and thought to wear it to the ladies' luncheon. *Kleider machen leute*, or maybe *unterkleider machen leute*.

The big day came, and I showered and dressed, put makeup on, clipped on some earbobs, and was ready to go, as always with me, running just a little late. I had agreed to pick up another guest and so zoomed downtown before heading up the mountain. In my excitement and nervousness, I hardly felt my clothes at all. The wind was in my hair. I made all the traffic lights and headed to Town Mountain Road. It was only when I parked the car and greeted our hostess that I realized something was amiss in the panty area. Cheek creep—the lacy bits had somehow been overwhelmed by the still-round bottom they were trying to contain. I was feeling very breezy at this point, in my flowing cotton skirt.

And I found that I liked it. Yes, the thong effect was rather pleasing, something I never thought to admit. I retired the size sixes for another day and went out a few days later and bought a thong. Cotton. Skimpy. Just the right thing, this thong. I've loved it in skirts, under pants, even in a business suit. Going bare—or commando, as they say—is also fine. But that thong (and the ones that followed) signaled a whole new world for me. The world of sexy undies. For those of you who actually know me, this may well qualify as Too Much Information. But somehow I don't think so.

A word about one of the loves of my life must be inserted here. If you do not have a massage therapist, ask all your friends for recommendations and find one. I like a massage once a month. Actually, I'd like a massage once a day, but Renee was named Best Massage Therapist by our weekly newspaper. She's moved into new quarters and is very busy. Also, this is her job, so money must exchange hands. She has given me an occasional free massage, but the girl's got to eat and buy cat food for the kitties.

But I digress. Find yourself a good masseuse. Or masseur, I'm not sexist about it. Establish a relationship with this person and then get naked. Do this now. Don't wait until you think your body is "presentable." Your body is gorgeous right now, and you will be so much happier when a professional like my darling Renee has oiled you and prodded and kneaded you like a mound of willful bread dough.

Renee always lets me choose a scent for the oil too. Sometimes I'm in the Georgia piney woods. Sometimes I'm all "rosemary for remembrance." One day, in the spring I think, I was lavender. There's some gentle music on, and her hands are warm, and I drift away from the sheer physical pleasure of it.

As I began developing and working this program, I was also in the early stage of menopause. That in itself has been quite an adventure, and I've considered a chapter here called "Willendorf at Midlife." As my estrogen levels fluctuated, my libido did the same.

I am now a woman of the Thirteenth Moon, for whom menstruation has ceased. In societies that don't value women unless they are breedable, women can be conflicted by this natural status. The road into this uncharted land is beset by legendary monsters, after all: hot flashes, mood swings, crashed libido, obscure cravings, gouts of blood. You must be a cunning warrior to wend your way through. You will need companions and allies.

But oh! When you reach that place—when you hold your wise blood—it is a time to rejoice. With herbs, some meds, a strong will and imagination, you can revive your flagging sex drive. With humor, you can reinvent your life and its purpose, if need be. It is a golden land here underneath the Thirteenth Moon, and your sisters stand ready to welcome you.

I began thinking about my own early esoteric exercise with Kundalini energy. I reviewed some of my old books and made a list of books I could consider to reconnect that part of my soul to the healthy glowing earth spirit inside. I looked forward to this part of my tantric work because reading is my favorite exercise.

Tantra comes from a Sanskrit root word "tan" which means to stretch, expand, weave, and manifest. In Western culture it has come to mean the study of sacred sexuality. I've recommended several books in the back, but the one I think best for starting out in the quest for uncoiling the snake-self is *Lady Chatterley's Lover* by D.H. Lawrence. I read it in college and loved all the juicy bits. But looking back at it from thirty years away, I found I couldn't remember how it ended. I now suspect that I never read the ending, only the juicy bits. So I corrected that injustice by buying a used copy and read it while riding the stationary bike.

The writing is very good, and the characters are beautifully drawn. I remembered the part where Connie laments her "slack belly" and how the girls gave themselves to their young German lovers right before the First World War. It was poignant and lovely. So start with that one. Begin to get a feel of being in touch with all your body's needs, not only the ratio of fruit to grain but the warm fuzzies of your sexual nature.

I am looking at a copy of *Cosmo* that I bought at the grocery store today. I also bought Portobello mushrooms, a bag of spring greens, a corkscrew, and a piece of poster board, all of which will likely be better for my sex life than this magazine. But this is the self-proclaimed "sexy" issue and features sexy haircuts and the "25 Sexiest Things Of The Year" and the Maxim Sex Files, whatever that is. So in the spirit of discovery and telling myself it's research (and because I am getting a haircut next week and need some ideas), I am spending part of Sunday morning reading a copy of *Cosmo*.

When was the last time you looked at this magazine? College for me, I think. Wow, is it an eye-opener. I know it's a tired joke, but a couple of the articles are good. There's a thorough update on safe-sex practices and birth control. Useful and certainly not taught in public schools as it was back in the day. But all the articles on sex—and they are legion—are, excuse me, lame. No new information, nothing interesting to a middle-aged woman who came to sexual maturity in the '70s. So I guess I'm on my own in this chapter. Wish me luck.

Speaking of the '70s, that was the time when we were willing to try just about anything. No, wait, it was anything. It was a golden age between the Pill and legalized abortion and the grief of HIV/AIDS. There was a kind of glorious abandon as we flung ourselves into a joyful new world of physical pleasure. We read the *Kama Sutra*, the *Joy of Sex*, *Oui*, Anais Nin. We imagined the smell of the sexy Paris streets, and we got hints about this Hindu thing called tantra. At least we thought it was Hindu. We knew it was about sex.

As near as I can tell, as it is filtered through my Western mind and after a year of moderate study, tantra is a series of exercises and meditations with the goal of integrating your personal Kundalini energy into your general life force. In America, we tend to think of sex as something outside life, not as the life force itself. As with bodies, we tend to have a skewed and perverse image of sexuality—we either revere it and remove it from daily life, use it to sell products, or we revile it and insist its only purpose is procreation. What if we thought of it as a physical expression of the dynamic energy that both is and runs the universe? Something healthy and healing and vital to keeping the connection we're building with the world we love?

Experts on tantric yoga and Eastern philosophy will have more detailed ideas of all this. And there are scores of books for those of you who want to go deeper and teachers with whom you can work. Some celebrities claim to have gloriously integrated lives due to their tantric work. All I know is, tantric exercises help me access my inner Sheela-na-Gig, and I'm including a few here as an appetizer for you.

I developed this first exercise when I was thinking about Sheelas and doing crunches on the floor. Crunches are boring, I confess, and my mind tends to wander. So I was counting, feeling the muscles and thinking about ancient Irish art.

You learned about the Goddess of Willendorf earlier in this book, our darling Willi. Another strong woman image that was prevalent in ancient art is called the "Sheela-na-Gig." Sheelas are found in lots of unexpected places, often in old churches, sometimes on stone columns. There's a worn one at Tara in Ireland, and I have a dark Sheela who sits on my altar.

She is not a delicate Goddess image, crowned in flowers, dressed in flowing robes. She is usually plain of face, stringy of body, butt-naked and grabbing her genitals. What's not to love?

After I've warmed up, done my crunches, stretched my legs, I lay prone on the floor and breathe deeply. When I'm ready, I raise my knees into the air, stretch my arms out to the sides, and continue breathing. I bring my arms down to my thighs, breathing into my legs and grasp the back of my upper thighs and let my legs drop to either side, as far as they can. As usual, breathing is key. As I breathe, I feel the energy moving through my body but originating in that root chakra. My knees come back up, still breathing, and I repeat the process several times. When my workout is finished, I feel deeply connected to my female roots. And I've had some great upper leg stretches.

Another exercise I do is to lie on my belly and breathe into the floor. I visualize my inner workings—ovaries, uterus, etc.—and imagine them connected to the world outside my body through my breath. I visualize the ovaries as trees, the uterus as a deep and holy well. I do this for five minutes or so and come away from the meditation very grounded and with a nice warm belly.

A long, warm bath becomes a tantric exercise when you light those candles, put oil in the water, and pour water over you as you bless your physical self. Watch your floating bits and remember how much water is part of your nature as an animal.

Pleasure is not a bad thing. Let me repeat that for emphasis. Pleasure is not a bad thing. In modern Paganism, we have this beautiful liturgical piece called the Charge of the Goddess, written originally by Doreen Valiente. One of the lines is—All acts of love and pleasure are My rituals. Pleasure as prayer is something so shocking to the Western mind that you may have recoiled from that line. But in this uncoiling chapter, we can touch on another aspect of loving your body and that is allowing yourself the thought of using pleasure as a sacred act, as prayer.

Pleasure. Say it aloud slowly. Pleasure. Now touch the tips of your fingers to your lips and slowly trace the outline of your mouth. Take a deep breath and repeat the process. Let your lips part and touch the tip of your tongue to one of your fingers. Extra points if you just ate a tangerine (as I did). Breathe slowly, letting the breath escape through your parted lips, warming your fingertips.

Sometimes pleasure—and our soul's and body's demand for it—is fierce and unrelenting. We want to be gripped firmly and pulled toward another body. The kisses then are wild and hard, the touch of hands on flesh frenetic, driven.

Sometimes our desire for the beloved smoothes all other thought from our minds, and we want to give ourselves over to pleasuring our partner, as a gift, as a love token. Our cousins, the bonobo chimps, have it right, gentling each other through touch and orgasmic delight.

Sometimes we want to take our time as we would with a meal in a fine restaurant. You have the whole afternoon and evening before you: you have given each other the gift of time. Slow down. Turn off your damned phones. Set the stage—have refreshments (water, wine, chocolate, snacks), toys, lubricants, condoms/dams, soft towels and moistened wipes at the ready. Music, if that works for you both. Good smells (incense or candles) if ditto. Take your time. Savor every morsel. Practice subtleties. Circle back around and try things again, either because they didn't work or because they did. Rest in each other's arms. Pee when you need to (really, don't hold it in). Feed each other. Laugh together. Touch each other in all the places that the beloved enjoys. Ask and receive. Experiment. Pleasure each other.

A local artist, who is passionate in all aspects of living, had recently gotten involved with someone she'd had her eye on for several months. They'd been out together for drinks and supper, for coffee and bagels. They'd stayed in together— sipping wine, sharing stories, delighting each other with simple facts about their daily lives, inspiring each other with visions of possibilities, as new couples have done since the beginning of time.

There came a weekend when their schedules meshed and the artist invited her kind friend to an old-fashioned sleepover at the artist's house. She prepared her guestroom with soft blankets and deep pillows, not assuming anything about the intention of the night. My goodness, what a sleepover it was. They were both bent on sweet and thorough seduction, and it was a perfectly lovely beginning to their personal love story. They listened to their bodies' desires and took time to explore all the possibilities.

As you can no doubt tell, I am an advocate for honest pleasure; given where I live you might even say I am evangelical about the subject. But I want to stress the word "honest" and add to it the word "honorable," and with those words we begin a never-ending, growingly nuanced discussion of consent. We never spoke of that when I was a young woman, and we seem to talk about nothing else these days. Let me be very clear about issues of consent and the right uses of personal power.

There is nothing wrong and everything right about verbally checking in with your partner or partners at every stage of engagement. If you don't have them already, add the following phrases to your toolkit for societal interactions.

How does that feel?

Thanks, love, but I don't enjoy that.

Right now, I'd love to_____. May I? Shall we?

Where would you like to start?

What would you enjoy tonight? What would give you pleasure?

If your partners say "no" or push you away, you are obliged to stop what you're doing. The more you engage in verbal clarity, the easier it all is. Don't trust your interpretation of someone's body language, and don't expect your beloved to read your mind. Ask, simply ask. Never assume you know the answer at this moment in time and in the relationship. Ask. "You liked this last time—shall we do that again?"

Never assume that your expressing your preference gives you carte blanche to expect that. Your partner or partners may express an academic interest but prefer to not participate at this time. I had a sweet lover who told me early on that he was indifferent to receiving oral sex, a technique with which I have some skill. When an appropriate time presented itself, I asked if he'd like to try it with me. He said he would, and we proceeded slowly. At every change in technique, I checked in with him. When I was ready to move on to other delights, he was happy with the experience. He said he'd never had a partner who was enthusiastic about oral sex, and that made a difference in his enjoyment of it.

When we are reluctant about particular techniques, that is not clean consent. Verbal conversation should accompany these forays into unknown territory. All of us have preferences for companionship, for refreshment, for all sorts of things. If you have pleasures and desires that your partners don't want to participate in with you, you have some choices to make. That is another set of conversations, mostly with yourself, about the nature of your needs and wants and the value of the relationship in which you are bound.

Consent is the first line in intimacy. Get used to talking about it sensitively and unequivocally. It is the key to pleasure for all of you.

We Pagans dream of a mythical and lustier time, of greenwood marriages and forest trysts. We linger on the words from Kipling's famous song of tree worship, "A Tree Song."

"Oh do not tell the priest our plight, for he would call it a sin, But we've been out in the woods all night a-conjuring summer in;
And we bring good news by word of mouth, for women and cattle and corn, For now is the sun come up from the South by Oak and Ash and Thorn."
[Kipling, R., *Puck of Pook's Hill*, 1906]

Because I am a creature of the early 1980s, I must also caution you about instituting safe-sex practices. If you are unsure what those are, please go to the website for Planned Parenthood. And heed what you read. Common sense can go a long, long way, but I do not always practice my wisdom protocols when all I want... right now... is hot, wild love.

Many years back, I was at a local Pagan festival with my teenaged Goddess-daughter. Her mother and I had waxed poetic about what would happen when she was ready to be sexual with someone. We talked about a warm summer night, the scent of flowers on the soft breeze, the pheromones that would make a potential partner smell delicious. I was sitting with friends around a fire when she scampered up to me, squatting down beside me to whisper in my ear. "He smells really good," is all I remember of that little conversation. But I know we spoke briefly. I reminded her about condoms (and where they were in the tent) and taking things slowly. She gathered her supplies from my duffle bag and galloped off into the twilight.

When my daughter was young, she asked me excitedly about the button in her yoni. When you touched it, apparently, it felt very good. Did I know about that? She seemed a little surprised that I did indeed know about the button and that most every woman has one. I am hopeful that it didn't diminish her pleasure in her discovery—pun intended—to learn that it wasn't unique to her.

As I grow older, as the Crone time approaches, I find myself adjusting to new expectations on my body, my libido. While I was transitioning into menopause, there were many long months of noninterest. Not in a partner, not even in my button. I began to talk to my contemporaries, and we traded some interesting observations about coming of age in the untamed 1970s, rearing children—especially girl children—in the age of HIV/AIDS and what it means to move beyond childbearing to a new land.

What do you say about a generation of women, many of whom came of age sexually during a period of time that has come to be called The Sexual Revolution? We heard the harsh strictures of our mothers—the only time they talked to us about sex. Dire warnings of what should or shouldn't be done, laced with a tinge of regret, spiced with a dash of longing for the freedom they felt during WWII, when the men were gone and the factory floors were filled by strong, happy women.

We reinvented the notions around women and sex, found ways to grapple with issues of intimacy divorced from issues of pleasure. Some of us learned that our affections and lust lay in other women, some of us discovered that serial monogamy was best, some of us discovered that we took love and pleasure where we could find it, and the gender of our partner mattered less than the connection.

The Roe decision gave us more choices, birth control options blossomed before us. There were toys and lotions and whispered talk of tantra. We licked honey from our partners' bodies and lay sated and alive. We read long-forgotten histories of how the world could be, how it was. There were blue curves of water and sandy shores, the smell of shellfish on our fingers. We were pioneers in a beautiful land.

Then the Reagan years fell upon us, and some of our friends grew ill and died from a new disease. The mood of the country turned cold, as we grappled again with who we were and how we were. Then Bush and Clinton and Bush. Sex-slave trafficking and Internet porn and women who call themselves feminists getting boob jobs. We stand now on the edge of a new territory, with the ravages of another land behind us. In that land, sexuality has become again a commodity, a terror, a point of pain and argument and grief. We dream of those heady days and nights when we were powerful and free.

Remember the France of Anais Nin's stories? The long nights, the frisson of excitement and desire? What if we had that now? At our age? With a dash of humor and a cupful of hope, the mystery of new lands to be conquered and enjoyed is good for our woman-souls, our woman-bodies. There will be honey in this new land and freedom and heat.

There are four adult stores in my area. One is a place to buy all sorts of gear. Two others are owned by the son of a former restaurateur here, and those stores are fairly standard video stores with toys to purchase and an "arcade" where one can pay an admission fee to watch films. One may also go to the arcade in search of fleshy and anonymous encounters. I have visited all three, had interesting conversations, and made interesting purchases.

The fourth is a much more genteel establishment, lovelier in every way. It is focused on an upscale female clientele who are looking for fine lingerie, delicate kink, and high quality toys. It is very posh and fun in its own way.

You can get anything you want on the Internet, but I prefer to handle the merchandise before buying. And there is a certain guilty pleasure about walking into a store and looking at all the merchandise. If you are an older, confident woman, you'll also see how the men react as you saunter into the place.

Toys can be great fun. I encourage you to explore them if you are curious. They can be used alone or with company, fun for you and your partners. You may be surprised to discover how much delight can be found in some vibrating latex, with or without a partner.

Blessed as I am with a circle of adventuresome women friends, shopping trips (for vibrators or corsets or underpants) are luscious excursions. We recently left the Goddess Temple in a giggling cluster, and I asked about personal lubricants. In an excited chorus, they responded with "coconut oil." I had been using it for ages as a drawing oil for my dental health and in the winter as extra protection for my face. But lube? It was an epiphany. And an example of how old dogs can be adaptable if the new tricks are as helpful as coconut oil.

CHAPTER 16

IT'S RAINING MEN

As someone said to me today—you look great, but I always thought you were beautiful. Isn't that sweet? I thought so. To be fair, I always thought I was kind of beautiful in my bodaciousness. But when your body comes more into line with what the culture deems acceptable, let me tell you, it's a whole new ball game. Part of it may be your renewed or newly discovered self-confidence. Or the fact that you have more energy. Or maybe you're feeling happier because your body is so healthy and alive and you smile more. I honestly don't know, but I'm not sure if I'm willing to give some of those folks the benefit of the doubt.

Either way, people are going to start noticing you in an entirely different way. Sad, but true. You go from being the girl with the pretty face and good personality to the woman with the sweet ass. I know, bizarre. But it happened to me, and it happened to others. Let's take a look.

I don't remember when it began exactly. Customers at the bookstore would comment on my changed appearance and say things like "good for you" or "you look nice." Then someone said, "When are you going to stop wearing those baggy clothes and wear something sleek and sexy?" My friends and coven mates would call me "hot." As a middle-aged woman prone to hot flashes, this seems somehow appropriate.

At Beltane that first year, I got my weight under two hundred pounds and I was feeling good. I'll tell you a little about this holy day, and I think it will seem familiar to you and most Americans.

Beltane is an ancient Irish holiday that is celebrated at the beginning of May. In fact, in Irish, the month of May is Bealtinne, which has something to do with bale fires. It is one of four fire festivals celebrated by many Pagans, and it marks the beginning of summer on the Celtic calendar.

Beltane is celebrated with dancing around the Maypole, bringing May baskets full of spring flowers to your relatives and friends, and drinking May wine. We wear flower crowns and flowing dresses, and we feast and dance and celebrate; though, to be honest, most Pagan holidays have a certain amount of feasting, dancing and celebrating. That's just how we are. Celebratory and experiential.

Is this sounding familiar? School children in our area of the South still do Maypole dancing and talk about faeries and May queens on the first of May. It's one of many ancient customs that have found a place in the modern world.

So here we are at Beltane. I had humiliated my daughter by making her (male) teacher a flower crown. He, in turn, humiliated her by actually wearing it for a while. We'd planned a lovely ritual of—yes, you've guessed—dancing and feasting for later in the evening. We'd invited lots of guests to join us—Beltane being a very friendly sort of holy day.

The male guests seemed particularly attentive. What in the world was going on? Lots of hugs, lingering glances, teasing comments. I am a friendly sort of person, and it is Beltane, after all. Everyone's a little flirty, a little tipsy. It turned out though that it wasn't just the holiday, it was my new body. Though we all enjoyed Dio's May wine with sweet woodruff, there was something more than usual going on.

And now my suspicions were confirmed, often with total strangers. Men on the street smile and flirt. When I'm stopped at a traffic light, drinking water, singing some bubblegum-music song on the oldies radio station, men in trucks hang out the windows to catch my eye. They make kissy faces or whistle or just smile and nod.

I despise it.

I'm a friendly person, Southern to the core. Raised right, with good manners supplied by my maternal grandmother, who was a city girl. My advice to you is to enjoy the attention (if that's your thing), but don't take it seriously. It will seem like you have a banner over your head:

Here's Someone Who's Building Some Big Self-Esteem: Welcome!

We explored the importance of consent elsewhere, but I will say a few extra words here on consent versus going-along-to-get-along. Clean and informed consent is the foundation for a rich life of physical pleasure. This requires you to know what you like, what you want to try, what you love, what you desire. If your partners want you to do something you find distasteful and you acquiesce, you are not being fair to yourself or to them. Examine why you'd give away your power or why you're squeamish. Tell your partner your reluctance and talk about it. We are living in a world where women have been owned, have been treated like the property they so often are. You have the right to decline without guilt or explanation. For some people, however, it is not safe to say "no." I ask you, if that is your situation, to find help in your community. Because a free woman is a sight pleasing to both see and be.

When new attentions are being paid to you as a result of your own hard work and self-love, you may find that you feel flattered or tempted or angry. I've felt all those emotions as I sort out my own feelings about my "new" body. I liked my body the way it was "before"—I liked my strong legs and round shape. So this new body is different, but I don't necessarily think it's more beautiful. And when people are trying to be nice and tell me how much younger or prettier or better I look, I try to be understanding, but sometimes it hurts. And sometimes it makes me mad.

Go ahead and feel what you need to feel about it. But please take time to figure out how you feel about your new shape, and don't let all those others determine how you feel about you. The way you feel may vary from day to day, so it's good to find ways to think about how you look, not just how you feel. Several years ago, I met a famous Pagan writer, a woman whose work I had admired for many years. I was invited to have dinner with her before her lecture, and she was warm and funny and personable. And she was large.

Beautifully large.

Patricia Monaghan had the kind of Earth Goddess juiciness that I thought was my own special magic back in my fat-woman days. Pat exuded self-confidence and female power in a way that says "Goddess" to those around her. Her talk and slide show about Ireland were inspiring, but it was her physical self that so impressed me, because her physicality at that time was the body I used to live in. And for the first time in a year, I missed it. I missed the fat glory that was me, and I felt great sadness that I couldn't be that woman ever again.

It took me some weeks to come to terms with the loss of that self. And it has taken even longer to come to terms with the loss of that wild Irish rose, Patricia Monaghan, who died in 2013. My world is smaller for her absence from it. I came to terms with both losses through writing in my journal and talking to my friends and remembering how hard it used to be to have the kind of energy that flows through this new me.

Patricia Monaghan was—and is—very beautiful to me. I hope she loved and appreciated that incredible body. But in the years we knew each other, we never talked about that. We spoke of Brigid, the difficulty of learning Gaeilge, the sorrows of the Irish diaspora—but never about her body.

As your body and your attitude both change, make sure to practice grounding and shielding. Have long chats with yourself about the juicy possibilities while being aware of your own preferences. Uncoil as you will and fill your sweet hands with sweet pleasures. What are your preferences? What are your desires?

JOURNAL NOTES

CHAPTER 17

EXERCISE—WAIT, I HAVE TO DO SOME RIGHT NOW

I believe in a previous chapter I expressed my general disdain for jocks. You may recall I was an artsy bookworm in high school, who reluctantly attended pep rallies and showed her school spirit by placing second in a sculpture competition at the state Latin club conference—with a clay model of indolent Bacchus.

I grew up poor in a rural area, so my options for athletic activity were limited to riding ponies and climbing hills and apple trees. If I had been interested in team sports, there was basketball. As a matter of fact, my high school had a pretty good girls team. But at five feet four, basketball was out of the question for me after I left middle school even if I'd been so inclined. This was before Title IX. There weren't many school athletic options for girls.

But sports didn't appeal to me the way languages, writing, theatre and the arts did. I sang in the chorus, did forensics league, Latin club, ecology club. Definitely not a jock. Now the tables are turned. Two of my close friends are, I'm sorry to report, jock-like. One was a competitive swimmer, a woman who now likes long, strenuous hikes and the occasional sweaty game of tennis. The other plays all kinds of games, seemingly for the fun of it. Frisbee, football, disc golf. Watches sports on TV. I am very fond of them both, but they are definitely jocks.

And guess what? I've become, if not a jock, at least amenable to exercise. It all started with a gentle walk around the neighborhood after I dropped my daughter off at school. Another mom and I would walk through this sweet, historic neighborhood and talk about life, school, parents. We walked a couple of miles, gently, a couple of days a week.

But as part of this program, as one of my Willi goals, I determined to walk every day. There's a nice park near my house, and I drop my daughter off at school and then take a walk before work. I started off with a couple of miles and went incrementally up to three miles. Each morning, I began the work of the day with this long period of thinking-and-stretching time.

I've seen this familiar park in every kind of weather and have been awed by the river in full flood and soothed by the river on a lazy day at the height of summer. I observe crows and geese and jays as they do their thing in the spring and fall. I've watched a beaver float down the river and a crawdad cross from a wet ditch to the stream.

Recently there was an unusual bird in the river, a bird I couldn't quite explain. It looked like a big duck, but something about the head was wrong. A man who wasn't a park regular came toward me as I walked, and he had a big smile on his face. "Did you see that? There's a loon in the river! Isn't that cool?" A loon in western North Carolina—yeah, I'd say that's pretty cool. The loon stayed on the river for three days, a feathery tourist from the lakes of the north. On its final day, it stretched its wings as though it was about to fly and arched its neck.

I invite people to join me sometimes, but mostly I walk alone and think and dream. Sometimes other walkers enter my space, and we walk together for a while, chatting, huffing and puffing. Generally, we don't know each other's names, but we smile and nod pleasantly, acknowledging our walking commonality.

There came a time when this solitary walk was not enough. I added a workout with three-pound weights a couple of times a week. That has expanded to four times a week, and the numbers of repetitions and exercises have grown over the months. I recently borrowed a five pounder but am being a little careful about what I do with that.

For my birthday, my family gave me an ancient blue bicycle, and I learned that skill again. I had two horrible bike wrecks as a kid, so maybe I should say I learned the skill for the first time. Though, to be fair, it's easy to wreck your bike on a dirt road. All my cousins did it too.

Sometimes in the morning I'd run for the sheer joy of doing it, walking part of the way, running over the small wooden bridges. My knees don't like too much running, so I only do that on grass when my spirit commands me to run. And I run flat out, like I did when I was a kid. I run for the exhilaration of it. I run because it's fun and I can.

At a recent festival, I caught sight of a friend I hadn't seen in several months. She looked tired (we all had a long drive to the camp) and was carrying two large cups of coffee, one for her and one for her husband. She didn't see me at first, so I sprinted down the dusty road toward her. Not a full-out run but a jolly canter-across-the-meadow sort of thing. I was rewarded with a big grin and a coffee-laden hug.

My sister-in-law and her family live south of Atlanta, and we visit them a couple of times a year. We try to spend almost a week there, enjoying their hospitality and their pool. I walk every morning with Bosco the Crazy Little Dog and swim in the heat of the day. In the evening we watch telly and sometimes play board games.

Early on, they had gotten a new recumbent exercise bike, and we all tried it out. It is very cool. It has a place to put your water bottle and a digital readout of how fast you're going and how far and how many calories you've burned. It is right in front of the biggest TV set I ever saw. I don't watch much TV, so I had the treat of Cirque de Soleil while I did twenty minutes on the bike. We bought one for home not too long after. A recumbent stationary bike, not a giant TV. We all use it, but I use it most of all.

I spent my childhood climbing trees and hiking hills, but as I became an adult and a city dweller, I lost touch with the feel and smell of being in the woods. I never realized how much I missed it until my friend Tim talked me into a "walk in the park" at Richmond Hill.

There were so many things to see—frogs, turtles, ferns, and fungus. There was a sweet little creek and a path that reached downhill and clambered over the railroad track to a bend in the river. I often go into those woods alone, armed with a backpack, a mango, and a bottle of water. I carry a walking stick, and my heart is light and joyful to be among the living and growing green things. It has reconnected me with a deep and important part of my essence that has long been hungry. I breathe in the rich air. I wash my face and hands in the ice-cold of the creek. It is the most glorious place and time.

What is that place in your life? The location that fills you with joy and connects you to the web of all being? Is it the high desert? Fifth Avenue? Skiing a snowy slope?

Let's try a short meditation to find your place in the sun.

Do your meditation preparation and give yourself fifteen minutes or so. Breathe deeply. Clear your mind.

CR80

You are sitting in a boat. You may decide the style of boat: a bass boat with a big Evinrude engine, a canoe from your favorite summer camp, a Viking longboat with a dragon prow. For me, it's a round coracle with one oar. You are now in your boat, leaving the shore, drifting into a strong current that takes you into the river.

The river is slow, safe, steady. You and the boat follow the current, and you notice the world around you. See the trees on the banks of the river. Notice the birds above you. Are there fish in your river? Other boaters? See the details in this world, as your safe passage is assured on the deep river.

Your boat begins to drift toward shore, and you see before you a little cove. Take up your oar now and gently guide the boat into the cove and onto the shore. Feel the earth as the boat is beached and then step onto the shore. A trail leads you into woodland near the beach, and you step on to the trail, heading inland.

The trail meanders among the trees, finishing in a promontory with a breathtaking view of the place you love. Drink it in—the sights, the sounds, the smells. Be specific in these things and try to see the actual place that your soul calls home. Are you looking over the ocean? A rich meadow? A village in Cornwall? The desert near Santa Fe? Own it, remember it, make it a part of your personal legend.

Now that you know, go there as often as you can. Make it a part of your life in a meaningful way. If it's far away, keep pictures of it around your house. Have bits of it (shells, stones, a vial of spring water from Kildare) wherever you are. Your soul will thank you. So will your kith and kin. Because when you honor your connection and love your body, you'll be amazed at how much fun you are.

And how much fun you have.

Fun. It's highly underrated in my life—how about yours? Do you find yourself getting all your chores done before you even think of doing something frivolous? And do your chores never seem to get done? Yeah, me too. There's always another load of laundry, there's always some dishes to wash, there never seems to be a day when there are no weeds in the garden.

Build in a little fun in your life. Remember how we found all those ways to love our bodies and to remember them to wholeness? Use some of those ways to bring fun—and with it, joy—into your life every day. Even something as simple as noting the color of the sunset and letting it take your breath away for a moment. Revel in this thing we call life. Don't put it off until your waist is a certain size or there's a particular number on the scale.

Be brave and fearless and embrace even the scary parts of your new body and your renewed life. See if the energy you have can be channeled into saving the world, loving your fellow creatures, and having some fun. The world won't end because you take yourself or your situation a little less seriously. At least I don't think it will. Why don't we all try it and see if the time-space continuum is altered at all? Let me know if your enjoyment of life somehow interferes with the planet's rotation, and I promise to do the same.

The summer I began my Willi work, I went to the beach with my circle of friends. We camped at an island off the coast of South Carolina called Edisto. I bought a new bathing suit for the occasion and used just enough sunscreen to prevent a burn but also let me get a "tan." I packed up the camping gear, shopped for some special food for my eating plan (peanut butter, crackers, fresh fruit), and hit the road in a van with three women, three children, and a standard poodle. Road trips—don't you love them?

The sea is one of those special places that makes me feel at one with the universe. My mountain family usually managed a trip to the beach in the summer where we roasted like lobsters, ate fresh seafood, and enjoyed the novelty of air-conditioning. I am neither a good nor a strong swimmer. I never had lessons as a kid, and as an adult I never had much interest. I could swim enough to enjoy a swimming pool and avoid drowning, but I wasn't a confident swimmer because I really didn't know how. I was an intuitive swimmer, I guess you could say.

My circle sisters wanted me to venture out with them "beyond the breakers." I carefully explained to these women who supposedly know and respect me that I wasn't a good enough swimmer to do such a dangerous thing. They laughed in my face. I stubbornly insisted that it was far too risky, and they let me be. They love me enough not to make chicken noises and flap their arms in my direction. At least when they're sober.

On the final day, two of them grabbed me by the elbows and dragged me into the water. They pulled and cajoled and got me out there. It was wonderful. And it was terrifying. But I felt one with the ocean, one with my friends, happier and braver than I'd been in years.

I also determined to take swim classes at the YWCA when I got home. I have had offers from folks who want to take me out in various boats—a sailboat, a kayak, a canoe—and it would be the worst sort of bad manners to fall overboard and drown during those charming outings.

I'm always on the lookout for new forms of exercise. I've asked a large friend of mine to teach me to throw a Frisbee and another friend to teach me to roller skate. I haven't done either one yet. But it's just a matter of time.

Along with the constant surprises of my changing frame, my interpersonal relationships surprise me too. My niece is very like me in appearance. In fact, when she was a girl, they sometimes called her "Byron Junior." She has blossomed into a tough young woman who knows her mind, and when I last saw her, we had a conversation that could never have happened even a year ago.

We were sitting in the living room, and she was telling me about her classes that semester and the four boyfriends she's currently juggling. We started talking exercise talk, and I found out she belongs to a health club near her work. And she has a personal trainer. A guy so cute she could "rip his clothes off with my teeth." This is an actual quote from my darling niece, spoken aloud in the presence of her mother, who laughed.

It got me thinking about the possibility of hiring one of those magical creatures. That may be the answer to some of these conundrums, all this searching my feeble mind for what my high school health teacher advised. But I've so far managed to avoid joining a health club or taking regular exercise classes (except for an irregular tai chi class), and I do take some pride in that. I work on my fitness in my living room, doing exercises like crunches on the floor and doing standing push-ups on our antique victrola. I do my tai chi form while listening to Loreena McKennitt, and I suspect it is becoming more dance-like than is strictly proper.

You don't have to buy a bunch of expensive equipment to get yourself in shape. You can take a walk and ride your bike and pick up a set of hand weights at a yard sale. If it will help you to stick with it to do classes with other people or have a personal trainer to keep you motivated, that's fine too. But it's not a requirement for good health that you spend a lot of money. You can pay in time, patience, and sweat, and that's a kind of currency we all have access to. Journal time.

JOURNAL NOTES

Try all sorts of exercises, all sorts of movements. Dance! Sing! Swim! Keep a list of what you like and what you don't. Play hard. Love big.

CHAPTER 18

I'm Waving Right Back At You—Loving the Parts You Can't Fix

Are you having fun doing this program? Have you found some extra time for joy in your life and have you learned—maybe reluctantly— to love your body? Yes?

Excellent.

The mom of one of my daughter's old friends— see how complicated relationships can be?—is also my friend. We've known each other since the kids were in elementary school, where we were willing volunteers, committee members, and penny counters. Early on in my Willendorf plan, Angie gave birth to the spectacular Noah, the only man I love. At a baby shower and blessingway in Angie's honor, a group of women came together to eat yummy things, cry a little, laugh a lot, and celebrate the motherhood of Angie and of all of us, as women are wont to do.

It was a hot summer day, so I wore a lightweight skirt and a sleeveless shirt. Many of the women hadn't been along on my Willendorf ride and were surprised to see less of me. I happily explained what I'd done and laughed as I wobbled my underarm flap at Robin. She returned the gesture with the line: I'm waving right back at you, baby! Let me know when you find the magic formula for this thing.

I was certain at that point in the process that it would take commitment and effort but I would—sooner or later—find a little less loose flesh hanging below my upper arms. I've checked all the triceps exercises I've heard of, and I do them fairly faithfully, at least three times a week. I've increased the number of reps. I've tried new postures. I've massaged and oiled and loved those dewlaps. If I push them up into my arms, I can feel muscles forming under there. I'm being patient and persistent and ever so hopeful. But sometimes I wonder if they will ever minimize, much less go away entirely.

Like the sadder but wiser moments when I hit the wall during my weight-loss adventures, I realized I needed a long talk with myself about this. I did what I've advised you to do—I got quiet, breathed deeply, made a still place in which I could listen to my deep earth self.

She was silent.

Hmmm. I scrunched down on the seat of the chair, breathed a few more times, thought beautiful thoughts.

Nothing.

Okay, what's up? I thought. Not speaking?

There was a gentle murmur from my deeper self, and I listened carefully, like someone hearing music from the house next door.

Slowly and quietly she emerged from her pool. And this is what she said: I thought you loved me.

It was the smallest voice imaginable.

I do love you. A lot.

But you hate your arms.

I don't hate my arms, I said firmly. It's just that they...

Aren't perfect?

No, no! That's not it at all. I revel in the power and glory of this machine. Perfection is the furthest thing from my mind. I'm only concerned with...

You are afraid to wear short sleeves in public, she said accusingly.

Am not.

Silence.

Okay, maybe I'm thinking that when these triceps have firmed up a bit, I can dig out those muscle shirts and wear them with some panache.

Why not now?

This time I was silent. For months I had been tackling the seemingly impossible tasks of losing weight, controlling my pancreas, keeping my cholesterol in check. I had cleaned out my wardrobe, walked in the foulest weather western North Carolina can offer. I had forgone chocolate and Guinness and ridden an exercise bike when all I really wanted to do was crawl under a blanket and sleep for a hundred years.

And my rewards had been strong muscles, boundless energy, and physical freedom. I was in love with the fantastic machine that was me, and we could do anything together, she and I. There was nothing we couldn't conquer, nothing I couldn't fix.

Here at last was something that might not be fixable, short of a plastic surgeon. Maybe I had lost too much weight and my older skin no longer had the elasticity it once had. These dewlaps, these signs of age and personal success, maybe they really weren't going away. And if they were not merely tourists but had taken up long-term residence, what then? Could I walk the walk and love them? Or was the Willendorf Woman a fake after all? Someone who can advise others to love their bodies no matter what but wasn't capable of doing the same for herself?

These arms are strong. They bend in all the right places. They have carried my child, buried my parents, risen in the predawn light of a solstice ritual. They are creatures of grace and beauty, soft as silk, pale in the best tradition of my British ancestors.

Remember Renee? While I was beginning to ponder this question, she invited me to take part in a workshop she was testing out, a workshop on exploring women's mysteries through the medium of massage. I wasn't sure what to expect but was up for time spent with like-minded women and maybe some massage.

I packed a small bag, a journal, a pen, some bottled water, and a few snacks since Renee had warned me it would be a day-long workshop. We started out with a guided meditation to get us in touch with our bird self, our sea creature self, and our spirit guide. We began with breathing—see, everyone does it—and I found myself slipping into a deep, peaceful place. I played around with being a peregrine falcon and then being a squid. I stepped lightly onto the interconnected web of all being, imagining the vibrating blue strings from an episode of *Nova* on PBS.

Then I stepped onto a new part of the web to commune with my spirit guide. This is always a powerful moment in a guided meditation. Renee's soft voice said, "You've come to your spirit guide with a question." Then she paused. And I blurted out to my spirit guide, "Do I really hate my arms? Are they going to be like this forever?"

That was not the appropriate question. Renee went on to explain that our spirit guide would help us design a massage ritual for each of us. I was bothering my spirit guide with some trivia about my triceps. Jeesh.

Renee went on to massage my arms, grasping me firmly by the wrist and working her way down those dewlaps. I felt the muscles underneath as she pulled and pushed and relaxed my shoulders. There was a kind of glory in those arms after all. I didn't need to pester my spirit guide about those triceps because, as we all know, the answer is in our hearts all the time. Renee noticed me smiling, I guess. But she was too wise to say anything.

Or maybe she figured she's a damn good masseuse. Which she is.

The same quandary is being presented by the saggy, baggy elephant skin on my inner thighs. I grasp the tops of my thighs—occasionally I ask total strangers to do the same—and I feel strength and barely concealed power. But those inner thighs... tsk, tsk. I am happy that my thighs no longer rub together when I walk, but the price I've paid for losing all that rich goodness is that the skin hangs in tiny ridges. Yes, I am walking. Yes, I am doing exercises that encourage development of those muscles. But like my dewlaps, it may be a question of too much skin stretched too tightly for a long time and now released. Maybe if I were younger, maybe if I had lost less weight, maybe if it had taken longer to lose it. Who know? Could be all the above. All I know is that my skin is saggy all over and I have the videotape to prove it.

During my fat glory years, people often thought I looked at least a decade younger than my chronological age. Customers in the bookstore were amazed to learn my real age. Those days are over. That luscious layer of subcutaneous fat is gone. The emergence of the Bone Woman signals the end of my perpetual youthfulness because as the fat gave way to bone and some muscle, the skin sort of... fell. I was interviewed by our local TV station last night on a Pagan-related matter. I wore a suit jacket, pulled my hair back in what

I hope was a professional do, put on a big beaded necklace and some lipstick, and worried about sounding like a fool. My husband videotaped my TV stardom, and I watched it the next morning. I sounded fairly sensible, for the which blessing, but I looked like... well, I looked like my mother. I looked like a woman every year my age. I didn't look fat (no double chin, no stubby fingers), but for the first time, I felt like I looked old. Okay, middle-aged may be nearer the mark, but the point is, I no longer look like a girl in the first flush of youth. Though my body youthens with every pound lost and every mile biked, my face is starting to show my age.

Now is the time where I put my money where my mouth is. I've poo-pooed all those vain folks who'll do anything to look young. I've mocked the current climate of doing anything to maintain a youthful appearance. But will I be able to look myself in the crow's-foot-festooned eyes and like what I see? Can the woman who embraced the Goddess as her body and honored its shape as it shifted from fat to fit adore the little wrinkles and sags that are the badges of a life well lived?

I discussed this with Dio just a few days ago. Years ago, I proposed that women should look for signs of wisdom on their faces. That little line near your nose that heads south toward the corner of your mouth and the line at the corner of your mouth that points north toward your nose meet to become a naso-labial fold. Imagine a world where we watch those lines carefully and call our best friend on the morning when they meet. With hushed tones, we discuss the implications of this ley line, this line of glory. We throw a little party, and we show it off to our younger friends who haven't quite achieved what we have. We are gracious in our croning, as we step into the birthright of mature female power. We are withholding the wise blood, and this intent is mirrored in our faces and bodies.

We can make that world. When we reach accord with our deep earth selves, we can bestow the gift of conscious aging on the next generation. It will take courage and strength to fly in the face of conventional wisdom. But you've done that in your walk with Willendorf.

Take the plunge with me. A new world—imagine that.

JOURNAL NOTES

Take time—either in your journal or in daydreaming—to imagine the world you want to create. How do people treat each other? How do they treat the natural world? Is there more art? More joy?

CHAPTER 19

THE THREE REBECCAS AND EXTREME MAKEOVERS

There are three incredible women in my life who are each named Rebecca. All three are called Rebecca but one—a friend from high school days—I call Becca because I have since high school days. Old habits and all that.

One Rebecca was a coworker of mine at the bookstore. I have known this Rebecca since my college days where we were both drama majors in a local university theatre department. She is about ten years older than I and has the most beautiful blue eyes ever. She's sassy and cranky and gloriously artistic. Rebecca the Artist is what I'll call her here to help you keep the Rebeccas straight.

The second Rebecca I've known for about fifteen years now, and she has moved from my town out to the West. She is a student of Santeria, Macumba, and Vodoun. She has long auburn hair, and she loves African dance and Latin music. She was married for a while to a man named Rolando but whom we called Johnny. She'll be Voodoo Rebecca for our purposes.

The third Rebecca is the high school friend that we will refer to as Becca. She is brilliantly creative and beautiful in the way of movie stars from the 1930s. We spent many an hour in our misspent youth trying to make our long hair stay in an up-do with one bobbie pin so that we could remove that single fastener and shake our heads for that tumble-down sexy effect. No, we didn't have those superlong bobbie pins, thank you very much. We had to use creativity and intuitive engineering.

Each of these women brings a special energy and light into my life and the lives of all the people they touch. Though they don't know it, each of them has become a mentor to me through this process. At various points, each one of them has appeared at exactly the right time to help me in ways I didn't even know I needed to be helped.

Rebecca the Artist reminds me of my deep and gnarled roots here in the oldest mountains in the world. We remember our town before it was the Taos of the East, when Asheville was a small city with a steady population and a quiet downtown. Rebecca the Artist inspires me with her bouts of mad creativity in which she dreams all sorts of businesses to start, including her dream of a flower farm in Tuscany. When we went to a movie featuring the glorious Tuscan countryside, we both had fantasies of different lives, far from our mountain roots.

Voodoo Rebecca mentors the wild side of me. She appears like a strange vision and talks to me like a shaman as she walks between the worlds of Anglo and Mexican, Pagan, and Catholic. She introduced me to the Festival of the Virgin of Guadalupe, and I went to our basilica to witness the most energetic Catholic worship I'd ever been part of. Music and babies and grannies and incense. I'm sure the Goddess at Guadalupe is very pleased with such joy and sound.

Becca is quiet and intense, a deep-eyed dreamer who lives in a perfect apartment with her elder dog Gracie. She is my comfort and my mentor in remembering that I can indeed be lovable. As a woman who loves through the world as a leader in my community, as a witch, as a priestess, I am pretty good about loving even the unlovable. Welcoming that love back into my being is a bit harder for me to trust. She never lets me forget how beautiful and talented and wise I am. I need that sometimes, to be honest. She mentors me through quiet evenings with excellent films and salade nicoise.

I hope you've gotten yourself some mentors while doing this program. You may have chosen folk with whom you could exercise or complain. You may have a food buddy whom you can call when the craving for a half-gallon carton of Rocky Road is too much to bear alone.

A mentor can be someone who actively supports you in your work with your deep earth self. And a mentor can also be someone who inspires you with their outlook or with the deliciousness of their daily lives. That's what the Rebeccas are to me. When I spend time with them—even electronic time on Facebook and Twitter, I come away with the desire to make my commitment to life deeper or broader or richer or fearless.

There is a woman whom I barely know who is an aging mentor for me. She works out at the local spa, talks about her pretty good, could-be-better diet. Her face has wrinkles that she sometimes rues. But there is a marvelous glow about her that may be attributed to a younger husband and a happy life and a couple of yoga classes a week. I'm not sure. When I see her, I want to glow like that when I'm that age. She makes me glad to grow older, to grow into my wise self, my crone self. And I am constantly seduced by the aging process of three of my favorite actors—Judi Dench, Helen Mirren, and Maggie Smith. Dames all, beauty in their experienced bodies and faces.

I have another mentor who I want to acknowledge here. Barbara is one of several people who are regular walkers down at the river park, people who come at about the same time each day that I do. She is in her late sixties or early seventies, and she is who I want to be when I grow up. Barbara is a widow, whose husband died just over a year ago. She says she won't remarry since she's buried two already. "Why would I want another man to wait on hand and foot?"

But she does have two boyfriends named Richard and a third potential boyfriend named Jeff, with whom she was having lunch the last time I saw her. Two of the men are younger than she, one of them much younger. The third is much older. All three love to go dancing, and Barbara may be the only person I know with enough energy to date three men who want to go dancing all the time.

For a while I called her "The Coconut Cake Lady" because I didn't know her name. Sometimes we walk together, and she is one of the best storytellers I've ever heard. She explained to me how she brings cakes to her doctor (who is also kind of cute) and that she had recently made a "Better Than Sex Cake." She outlined all the ingredients, and it did sound pretty good. But my favorite Barbara story has to do with those frozen coconut cakes you get at the grocery store.

Coconut was my late mother's favorite cake, and we still take a slice of it to the cemetery at Samhain and again on her birthday. So when Barbara started talking about coconut cake, my ears and taste buds pricked up.

She was going to get herself one of those coconut cakes at the store, and she was going to eat it, she told me forcefully as we walked the river track one day. She loves them (though she says the Better Than Sex cake is better), and they were on sale. She was going to leave the park that very morning, go to the store, and get a cake. Maybe she'd share it with her friends or her cute doctor, but maybe she wouldn't. She'd been watching her waistline, and she looked pretty good, I thought. She thought so too. The coconut cake began to assume epic importance.

When I saw Barbara a couple of days later, I asked about the cake. Haven't had time to pick one up, she said, but I'm going to get me one today, as soon as I leave here.

A few more days passed before I saw her again, and she still hadn't acquired the cake. After the weekend, I saw her heading my way on the track. "Don't say nothing about that cake," she exclaimed. Okay, my lips are sealed, was my answer. We walked for a few minutes in silence.

I worked up the courage to ask, "Did you finally get one?"

"One?" she practically crowed. "No, ma'am, I did not get one." I waited. "I got two! And I ate both the damn things! At my age, you've got to take the pleasures you can."

Barbara is a wild young soul in a wild old body, a body she cares for through attention to what she eats and a commitment to getting her walk in, sometimes twice a day. She uses her walk for exercise and also for therapy. Her late husband died after a long illness, an illness in which she tended him. After he was gone, she'd come down to the park anytime she felt lonely and take a long hard walk. Those endorphins blessed her as they do all of us, and she felt better. She also lost weight, firmed up, and sent her self-esteem level into the stratosphere. She is one of the coolest women I know, a real role model for me about the powers and virtues of positive aging. She and Mary Green are the two women I want to be when I grow old.

Mary Green was a customer at our bookshop, as well as a friend. She died last year after a rich life, well lived. She used to have a big magnetic sign on the back of her car that read "Be nice to me—I'm old." But it kept falling off. I remember her leafing through a makeup primer in the shop. "Just as I thought," she said, closing the book in disgust. "Nothing in here about how to make older skin look its best. I don't want to look like a thirty-year-old. I want to know what to do to have the best skin at my age." I didn't ask what that was. She was a beautiful woman, late '70s maybe.

And she had a valid point. Why can't we see more articles, books, and information about how to be the best-looking we can be at every age? The whole beauty industry is geared to twenty- and thirty-year-old faces. No wonder people are tucking and slicing and toxing their faces, frantically trying to be forever young. What do you do with wrinkles and sags? What kind of moisturizers does older skin need? Beats me. I use calendula oil that is compounded by a local herbalist. And I scrub my face with a soft brush, as my grandmother did.

I remember having a fancy once about aging, a fancy I outlined for you a little earlier. In my fancy, I carefully watched the line forming at the edge of my mouth and the accompanying line forming at the edge of my nose, like stalactites and stalagmites, joining at last to become the perfect naso-labial fold. You'd tell your friends about your wisdom line, and they'd be jealous because theirs hadn't quite connected yet.

Wisdom lines indeed. People spend perfectly enormous amounts of money to be planed and perfect, why would they want to have wisdom lines? Wouldn't that make you look old?

Heaven forbid.

While I was developing the Willendorf program, there was a show on a major network that featured ordinary folks having extraordinary plastic surgery. Now some of those folks really needed help—they required reconstructive surgery following a bout with cancer or a terrible accident. But some of them were just homely, out-of-shape, overweight people with no real fashion sense and no noticeable self-esteem.

Those folks spent months away from their friends and families. They were sliced and sucked and planed and finally revealed in their "new" bodies. Sometimes there was a big difference; sometimes they looked like they'd gotten new clothes and a haircut.

A lot of those people made me sad. They couldn't seem to start living because they weren't a size four or their nose was crooked or their teeth weren't white enough. I wondered why we keep doing this to ourselves, why we hate the thought of getting old or fat or grey-headed. Is it because we're so afraid to die that we think we can avoid it by staying young? Doesn't it sink into our psyches at some point that young people die too? Is it really a question of mortality, or is it, again, our painful disconnection from the material and earthly parts of ourselves? I guess by now you know what my answer is. I'd like to do one of those makeover shows and have those folks eat right and get some simple exercise, have them do some guided meditations, some breathing, and a whole lot of loving.

It wouldn't be an instant transformation but an ongoing process, a joyous ride to a sustainable, better life. Sure there'd be bumps along the way, a wall or two to hit, you might even fall off the wagon and have to love yourself back into shape. Kind of like you're doing. Good for you, by the way.

CHAPTER 20

WHY WE WON'T END UP IN THE NATURAL
HISTORY MUSEUM IN VIENNA

It has been more than a decade since that initial
weight loss, and I continue to go up and down
a bit. I'm not fearful of failure anymore and try to
be sensible about variations in weight and diet,
about what I eat and drink, all of it. There are
many new friends who never knew me at two
hundred and fifty plus pounds. When I refer to
myself as "fat," they can't imagine my large and
luscious former self, and when they see photos of
my '80s hair and my '90s figure, they shake their
heads in wonder. I do too, to be honest.

All this is my way of saying that you can do this
loving-your-body thing. You can do it now, and
you can stick with it. Yes, there will be difficult
times and confusing times. But if you listen to
yourself in love and with a bit of humor, you can
make this a long and beautiful road. If you start
this young, you'll have processes in place for the
changes that aging brings. If you start when you're
older, you have the same advantage. Embrace

your Willendorf now and reap the assurance and grace of a life deliciously lived.

I lost more than a third of my body weight that first year. People who watched my progress as the incredible shrinking Byron grew bored with my constant chatter about olive oil and the fascinating conversations I have with my deep earth self. But they love me and are proud of me and some of them are—bless them!—inspired enough to begin the same process by simply loving their bodies.

Even after all this time, all this talk, all these examples, I find it hard to believe that something as simple as finding a way to love your body has wrought so many positive changes for so many people. Who could have known that so many of us carried around a burden so heavy and so unnecessary? Years ago I took a women's spirituality class, and when we got to the section where we talked about our bodies, those freethinkers simply shut up. They couldn't go on with the spiritual and intellectual exercise that was the class because they were so afraid of even talking about their bodies. As I've said before, I must be a slow learner. With that example in front of me, I never guessed that there are so many people who so loath the very earthiness that sustains them.

No more, my dears. My eyes are at last open. I've embraced the Willendorf of my gorgeous and powerful body, and there is no turning back for me. And, I suspect, there will be no turning back for you.

When I was thinking and writing so much about the Goddess of Willendorf—the dear girl we've dubbed "Willi"—I wondered where she is now. Like a college roommate you've lost touch with, I worried a bit about this famous round girl—and so I did a Google search. She's in the Natural History Museum in one of my favorite cities in the world: Vienna.

I was only in Vienna once, when I was seventeen. It was romantic and eerily beautiful. The ruling Hapsburgs had a penchant for creepy funerary marbles, and those monuments are everywhere in the old city. There were also marvelous restaurants and wine bars, parks with Strauss waltzes played by small orchestras. I remember eating fresh cherries from street vendors and trying valiantly to buy an eraser in an art supply store. Vienna is the reason I became a German major in college.

But I digress. This is where our Willi lives—in the Natural History Museum in that exciting European city. I hope to go there one day and do homage to her in her exhibit. Until then I will love her from afar and love her image as it lives in reproductions in many sizes and media.

The Goddess of Willendorf is a potent symbol of human power, from a time when marketing people didn't define our notions of beauty. After all these years, her faceless head and still, heavy form speak of the awe—the reverence—

our ancestors must have felt for fertility and the powers of creation.

We will not end in the Museum in Vienna, my friends, carved from limestone, worn smooth from the touch of many hands. Though if your choice is to be touched smoothly by many hands, I am with you on that. But we have other fish to fry, as we say in the South, embracing ourselves as we really are and denying, once and for all, the societal and cultural voices that separate us from our deep and earthly selves. There is a new voice for each of us to hear, a voice we have long denied and ignored. We have heard the song of connection. We have been the Bone Mother.

Are you finding yourself smiling as you have these internal conversations with the deep part of yourself that is your real self? I feel a little sheepish sometimes. But I also am empowered and centered and whole, as though I made a pilgrimage to a holy well and found such love and peace in that ancient sacred place that I chose never to leave it.

I carry that peaceful place within and around me at all times, as I know you do. We have found a place for self-knowledge and self-appreciation that has long been denied us as we grow and age and change. We are all better for being aware of the connections between us and all the dancing atoms that make up our universe.

Enjoy, my dears. Stretch your joy and good health throughout your community and all your kith and kin. Be obnoxiously happy in your personal universe, and let the ripples of your joy open up cans of personal responsibility on the asses of those around you.

And don't stop those quiet conversations with the earthy self that you've come to cherish. As you walk or bike or stand on the bank of a river, keep reestablishing this all-important connection. Loving this deep self and honoring that love through listening may be the most important part of embracing your own Willendorf. As we go about the business of creating a new life in our healthy, happy, and altered bodies, keep listening, keep breathing.

I want to leave you with one final guided meditation, one of my favorites, something I've been doing myself and guiding groups through for many years.

You know what to do. Let the dog out. Put the music on. Go to the bathroom. Dress in your comfy clothes. Get your blankie and pillows and make yourself at home on the floor. As always, if it helps you to read the exercise into a little recorder and play it as you meditate, feel free. Or if you have a friend who has a beautiful voice, have them do it.

ℭℬ℘

Now breathe. Yes, breathe. Deep, earth-connecting breaths that vibrate the air around you. Fill your lungs and your blood and your being with the world around you. Let that mingle with your essence and return it to the universe. Again. Belly—remarkable bellows of the remarkable machine—rising and falling as you center yourself, your spine gratefully supported by the floor beneath you. Breathe with your hands on your diaphragm and feel yourself relax. Can you sense the expectation? Where are we going today? What will we find? And breathe.

Close your eyes and imagine that you are sitting in a cozy chair by a fire. I imagine a turf fire and a pint of Guinness. You imagine the fire and drink of your own choosing. As you drink the last of your beverage, feel the wetness in your throat, feel the cells of your body respond to the healthy hydration you have chosen today.

Rise from your chair and stretch like a cat. Yawn if you like. Feel your muscles flex and relax. Notice your surroundings. Take in the detail around you. What the walls are made of. What color they are. What's on the floor.

Walk to the door and let yourself through. Feel the texture of the door under your hand. Outside, the world is pleasantly warm, and the sun hangs low on the horizon, casting long shadows in your yard. Breathe. Walk down the path and out the gate, following a trail through the fields, a trail that was begun in the long-ago time.

Take your time as you walk, noticing flowers in the grass, and insects, maybe a deer at the edge of the field. You are heading toward the woods and you are going to meet someone there. That someone is your deep earth self, the person you've been conversing with this whole time. Finally you will meet, face-to-face.

Enter the line of trees. Notice their kind. Are they deciduous or evergreen? Old or young? Breathe the air in this new place. Breathe. Breathe. Your feet follow the path to a clearing in the woods. The sun is setting; the sky in the west is bright with the colors of twilight. At the edge of the clearing, stop and look around you. You are alone except for a standing stone in the center of the clearing. Wait in that place only moments as the sun sets and the moon rises. Breathe. Breathe.

If you remember your song, sing it now, in this place. Sing the song that connects your delicious machine to everything around it. Remember yourself as the whole, powerful, remarkable animal you are. Sing, my dear. Breathe deeply and sing.

You sense a stirring ahead of you and step out into the clearing. From behind the stone steps, your earth self is holding a gift for you. Walk toward each other until your deep self reaches out and puts the gift into your hands. You look down at the gift as your deep self retreats to the stone, always there, always waiting.

Turn and walk slowly back down the path that leads homeward. Through the trees. And breathe. Into the fields. And breathe. Under the moon. Breathe.

You reach your gate and raise the latch, entering your yard. Holding the gift, open the door and go sit by the fire again. Breathe. Stretch.

Look at the gift in your hands and remember that you are forever connected with the dancing elements that surround you and are you. When you are ready, open your eyes.

What was your gift?

THE WITCH'S TEST
KITCHEN: EATS AND SUCH

Long ago, a local chef approached my boss at the bookstore and asked for help in self-publishing a memoir/cookbook. Somehow I ended up editing the darn thing, which was a labor of love that was ultimately very rewarding. When I realized that I spent many words on what to eat and what I eat, I thought it might be fun to add some recipes to the back of this quirky little book.

These are in no particular order and are generally easy to do. Feel free to add and subtract ingredients you particularly like. I've tested them all and still eat them often. Except for the final two entries which I suspect I will never eat again. You'll see why when you get there.

I recommend homegrown and organic produce and meats for maximum nutrition and a minimum of toxins. Yes, you can substitute conventionally grown products, and your budget may require you to do so. No judgment, all love.

Romaine Salad with Nuts

If you can't eat nuts, leave them out. They are an easy source of extra protein, have few carbohydrates, and add richness and texture to all kinds of dishes.

Ingredients:

1 head of Romaine lettuce
1/2 C walnuts or almonds
1 T chopped garlic
Handful of baby carrots, chopped
1 small tomato, chopped
2 stalks of celery, chopped

Chop the lettuce into bite-size pieces. Clean if required. (I have a busy salad spinner, and I recommend them. Buy new at any kitchen and most department stores. Or pick up a lightly used one at a thrift shop.) Throw all the other ingredients into a large bowl. Add in the clean and spun lettuce. Toss with a large spoon. Eat naked or dress as desired. My preference for dressing is:

1/2 C cold-pressed extra virgin olive oil
1 t chopped garlic
1/4 C feta cheese
1 T apple cider vinegar
a few leaves of fresh basil, chopped
smidge of salt
grind of pepper

Whisk together everything but the chunky bits (feta, garlic and basil), then add those in and stir with a fork. Drizzle—don't drown your salad.

Spring Greens With Balsamic Dressing

Ingredients:

Spring greens (arugula, mesclun, baby spinach, little lettuces)
Hard-boiled eggs

Clean the young greens and take them for a spin. Slice the hard-boiled eggs into even slices—I also like to chop up one of eggs and toss it in the greens.

Balsamic Dressing Ingredients:

1/2 C cold-pressed extra virgin olive oil
4 T. balsamic vinegar

Get the best quality balsamic vinegar you can find. Whisk these two perfect ingredients together and toss your greens with them. Arrange the egg slices on the top of the salad. Consider a wee glass of Châteauneuf-du-Pape.

Hannah's Celery Logs

Hannah is now a grown woman, but when she was a little woman, she used to make these for the children in our coven on meeting nights. The adults liked them, too, and often gobbled them down before the little ones did.

Ingredients:

celery
peanut butter
dried currants

I always choose a no-sugar peanut butter, no preservatives variety. You can also use almond butter or cashew butter. You should not do this if you have a nut allergy. Obviously.

Clean the celery, remove the strings along the ribs. Cut it into two- to three-inch lengths. Stuff the nut butter into the crevice. Dribble the dried currants or small raisins along the top of the nut butter. Arrange carefully, with olives to garnish the plate. Big fat black olives or those olives preserved in oil. Hey, or maybe those big green ones with garlic stuffed inside. Anything the adults will go for first so that the kids can have their celery treats.

If you can't do the nut butter, try cream cheese. And sprinkle with teeny capers.

~~~~~~

TOFU AND BROCCOLI IN PEANUT SAUCE

Ingredients:

1 block of firm tofu, cut into ½" cubes
1 head of fresh broccoli
¼ C peanut butter
1 T chopped garlic
splash of soy sauce
1 T olive oil (to sauté tofu)

Break or chop the broccoli into bite-sized pieces and steam it until tender. Drain it in a colander and set aside. Warm a large skillet and add the olive oil. Chop or crush the garlic and add it to the oil. Bring the heat up on the skillet and sauté the cubed tofu in the olive oil until it is crisp and golden brown on the outside. Remove the tofu from the oil with a slotted spoon and let it drain on some paper towels, reserving pan juices.

Set the tofu aside. Put the peanut butter in the warm pan with juices and whisk. You may need to add a little water to make the gravy. Simmer gently until smooth. Now add the broccoli and tofu to the peanut sauce, put in a splash of soy sauce and toss gently. If you have peanuts or walnuts, you can throw in a handful of those, too. Serve piping hot with brown rice and slices of blood orange.

CHICKEN BREASTS WITH ALMONDS AND FRESH GREENS

Ingredients:

4 boneless chicken breasts
3 T olive oil (to sauté chicken)
2 cups greens (spinach, collards, arugula, kale—you choose the ones you like best)
1/2 C almonds

Slice breasts diagonally into half-inch thick slices. In a large skillet, warm the olive oil and add in the fresh garlic, cooking until the garlic is beginning to brown. Turn the heat up and fry the chicken slices in the oil until they are cooked through. Set them aside, draining on paper towels. Add a little white wine or water to the pan juices and dump the cleaned greens into the pan. Stir constantly until the greens wilt. Return the chicken slices to this mix, lower the heat and simmer covered for 5-7 minutes.
Serve with fresh green beans.

Fresh Green Beans

That's all, just green beans

2 pounds of fresh green beans (come on, get organic ones)
smidge of salt
grind of pepper
1 T olive oil

Break the ends off the beans and snap them into smallish pieces. This should be done while talking to a good friend and drinking iced tea. Rinse them. Put them in a big kettle with cold water. Boil until just tender. Add the salt, pepper and oil. Simmer for five more minutes.

Collard Greens

Ingredients:

Two bunches of fresh collard greens, washed and chopped
3 T rendered pig fat (bacon or ham are good choices)
Smidge of salt

Fill a big pot with fresh water. Bring it to a boil and add the salt. Chop the collards and wash them thoroughly—they can be dirty little freaks. And when you chop the greens, set aside the thick stems and toss them into the boiling water first. It'll take them a little longer to get tender. After a couple of minutes, add in the leafy parts of the collards and stir them down as they boil. Lower the heat and simmer the greens until tender. Once the boil has become a simmer, add in the pork fat. If you don't eat pork or don't want that sort of fat, substitute olive oil. But honestly, ham juices or bacon drippings sure do flavor collards something fine.

LENTILS WITH SUN-DRIED TOMATOES

Ingredients:

1 C dried lentils
2 C water or vegetable broth
¼ C sun-dried tomatoes

Bring the water/broth to a boil and add the dried lentils. Lower the heat to simmer and cover the pot. Add the dried tomatoes and cook the lentils until they are tender. You may want some salt or some soy sauce or a little tamari or maybe some Bragg's Liquid Aminos.

PUMPKIN BUTTER

Every October, an astounding range of squash and pumpkins appear in every nook and cranny, waiting to be transformed into strange and hideous lanterns. I always grab a few of the small pie pumpkins and cook them into pumpkin butter. It needs to cook down for a long time and the house smells good during the process. Cleaning the seeds and roasting them gives you a bonus treat.

Ingredients:

1 medium pumpkin
1 C sugar
1 T cinnamon
1/2 T nutmeg
1/2 T allspice

Clean the strings and seeds from the pumpkin and peel off the thick skin. Retain the seeds. Cube the pumpkin flesh into chunks and place in a large kettle with a little water. Add sugar and spices. Cook on a low temp until the pumpkin is soft and the color has become a darker orange-brown. Puree it in a blender or food processor and return to kettle. Simmer another ten minutes or so until the flavors blend. Serve with toast points or biscuits. It is also good stirred into thick yoghurt.

Rinse the seeds and remove the strings. Put them in a bowl and drizzle a little olive oil on them, then sprinkle them with a little coarse salt. Toast the seeds in the oven at 350 for about ten minutes.

Apple Crisp

Filling:

6-8 apples, peeled, cored, cubed
1/2 cup sugar
1 T cinnamon
1 T nutmeg
pinch of salt
1 T flour
splash of soy milk or cream

Pick an apple you love—Cortland, Fuji, Granny Smith. I am fortunate to live in a region that grows good apples and my favorite varieties are Arkansas Black and Winesap. Peel and chop the apples and toss them with the spices and sugar and allow them to rest for 20 minutes. Toss them with a big spoon and add the flour, salt and splash of cream. Another good toss and a rest (about five minutes), then put them in a baking dish.

In the same bowl the apples slept in, make some topping for the crisp.

~~~~~~

CRISP GOO TOPPING

Ingredients:

1 C oatmeal
1 C granola
1/4 C olive oil
1 T nutmeg
1 T cinnamon
1 T allspice
1 C warm water

Pour all the dry ingredients into the bowl and fluff them by hand until mixed. Add in the olive oil and water, and work the goo into a fine mess. Plop it onto the apples and arrange it to cover the apples completely. Drizzle a little more olive oil onto the top and slide into a preheated 350 degree oven. Bake until the apples are soft and the topping is crisp, about 45 minutes.

~~~~~~~~~~~~~~~~~~~~~~~~~~~~~~~~~~~~~~

Pesto

Basil pesto is one of the greenest and sexiest foods on the entire planet. There are many kinds of basil but the best one is the one growing in your own garden. Bring it in warm from the sun and rinse the spider bits off it. Take only whole and perfect leaves, pinching out any flower heads that may be forming. The smell is intoxicating.

Ingredients:

3 C fresh basil, packed
1/2 C olive oil
handful of pinenuts or walnuts
big pinch of salt
1 T lemon juice
1 T chopped garlic

Put it all in the blender and puree. If it feels too thick, add a little water and puree till smooth. Serve with bread or over pasta or—my favorite—eaten with a long-handled spoon directly from the blender. Reminds me of my Daquiri days, I reckon.

~~~~~~~~~~~~~~~~~~~~~~~~~~~~~~~~~~~~~~

Poached Salmon With Dill and Garlic

This recipe can be used for any fat and delicious fish—trout, tuna, monkfish. Poaching is easy and gives flavorful and tender results. I also recommend doing fish en papiotte, which is all these ingredients (without the water) wrapped in a parchment paper packet and baked in the oven. Fresh, tasty, satisfying.

Ingredients:

salmon steaks
1/2 C water
2 T garlic
1/4 C dill, chopped

Poach the steaks in the water until firm. Remove them from the pan, and add a splash of olive oil to the remaining water and fish juice. Toss in the bruised garlic. Stir the liquids together and return the fish to pan, making sure to coat the steaks thoroughly with liquids. Simmer for a minute or two, then remove the pan from the heat. Before serving, toss the fish with fresh dill.

Baby Bella Soup

My great niece is named Bella, and when I clean these grubby little mushrooms and get them ready for a dish, I often think of her grubby little baby face. She is growing into a wondrous young woman now, but the dirty little baby mushrooms are as filthy as ever. Wash them, brush them, treat them with tough love, and you will be rewarded with their tender, plump delights.

Ingredients:

1 lb small portabella mushrooms, cleaned and sliced
2 quarts of vegetable stock
1 C spinach, chopped
1 T garlic, minced
2 T olive oil
Seasonings to taste.

Begin with the olive oil in the bottom of a warming stock pot. Add the garlic and bring to a simmer, stirring it occasionally. Then add the sliced bellas and let that simmer together until the mushrooms are tender. You can certainly make your own vegetable stock, and I encourage that. But when I was working the Willendorf program, I bought cartons of organic vegetable stock and used that. Either will do, depending on your inclinations. When the bellas are tender, add in the fresh spinach, allowing it to wilt in the warm oil. You are now ready to add the stock and pour it in carefully. Bring the whole thing to a stout boil, then reduce the temperature and simmer for about ten minutes. Serve with shavings of hard cheese, like parmigiano.

Broiled Bread with Olive Oil and Asparagus

Ingredients:

1/2 pound young asparagus
1 baguette, preferably whole wheat
4 oz. grated white cheese (not mozz)
minced garlic
olive oil

Steam the asparagus until it is bright green and just tender. Set it aside to cool a bit. Slice the baguette into one-inch wide slices and arrange them on a baking sheet. Drizzle the bread with olive oil and spread some of the minced garlic over that. Cut the asparagus into pieces about three inches long and arrange a few of them on each slice of bread. Add a splash of grated cheese to the top of the asparagus and place the baking sheet under the broiler for several minutes, until cheese is melted and bread is golden. Serve immediately, but try not to burn your fingers or the roof of your mouth.

~~~~~~~~~~~~~~~~~~~~~~~~~~~~~~~~~~~~~

Fresh Dates With Brie

Ingredients:

Medjool dates, as many as you can afford
Full fat Brie, real Brie, from France Brie

Pit the dates, lovingly. Split each one by pulling the sides away from each other with your fingers. Do this slowly. Suck your fingers when you've finished. Stuff each fig with a dollop of Brie. Mash the sides back together to secure the precious cargo, after which you can suck your fingers again.
You may broil them, if you like, but they are best eaten at room temperature, with a glass of good Prosecco and someone you love.

~~~~~~~~~~~~~~~~~~~~~~~~~~~~~~~~~~~~~

Chicken Stew

A perfect food. As we discussed with the vegetable broth, you can shorten the prep time on this by picking up a pre-cooked rotisserie chicken at the grocery store.

Ingredients:

A small whole chicken
3 C chicken broth
A small onion, chopped fine
Three stalks of celery, diced
A head of garlic, cleaned and chopped
1 C of baby peas

1 C diced fresh carrots
Salt, pepper, lemon pepper, oregano to taste

Cook the chicken in a stock pot in fresh water until cooked through. Allow it to cool in the water until it can be handled. Remove the meat, retaining the carcass and skin. Return these to the pot and add the onion, celery and spices. Return to a low boil and cook for thirty minutes. Why not have a glass of sweet tea and some cubed cheese while the stock does its thing? Chop the meat into bite-sized pieces. When the stock is ready remove the carcass, celery and onion. Strain the broth and return to the stove, adding the chopped meat, carrots and peas. Allow to simmer until the flavors have begun to combine.

~~~~~~~~~~~~~~~~~~~~~~~~~~~~~~~~

DIOTIMA'S MAY WINE

May wine is part of many Beltane celebrations and is a simple, delicious treat.

Ingredients:

German white wine
Fresh sweet woodruff
10 perfect strawberries

Add the cleaned sweet woodruff (a good handful) to a half-gallon sized glass canning jar. Pop in the clean, capped and whole strawberries. Now pour a bottle of German white wine (Zeller Schwartz Katz or Liebfraumilch) into the jar. Shake gently and refrigerate.

~~~~~~~~~~~~~~~~~~~~~~~~~~~~~~~~~~~~~~

GRIT TARTS

I created this for a book event for one of Charles Price's historical novels. I was attempting to create Breakfast in a Bite and this is what worked.

Ingredients:

I C coarse ground grits, prepared
¼ C grated cheese, your choice
½ C chopped mushrooms, your choice

How to prepare grits that are edible—follow the directions on the bag for the amount you want. Boil the water first, then add the dry grits. Depending on the grind of the grits, they will cook quickly or they will cook for half an hour or so, on a low temperature in a covered pan. Grits should not be runny. They should be strong and stout, ready to be a breakfast cereal with cream and honey. Or they will have shrimps and peppers and cheese. These are a staple food of the American South and we are particular about how they are served.

As the grits cool, they will become remarkably firm. While still pliable, press the grits onto the edges of a muffin pan, the kind for mini-muffins. You are making a grits crust. Allow it to firm up.

Sauté the mushrooms in a little butter until they are cooked through. Allow them to cool and then add dollops of mushroom into the center of each little muffin. Sprinkle grated cheese on the top. Use a butter knife to loosen each little muffin and place them on a pretty plate. You may garnish with fresh berries. Eat them when the heat of the mushrooms has melted the cheese.

Kayla's Trout, Avocado, and Goat Cheese Snacks

Ingredients:

Smoked trout
firm goat cheese, sliced thinly
avocado, sliced as above

Smoked trout is very sexy. Open the package and spread the trout on a small plate, breaking it into smallish pieces. Use the avocado slice as the base of your snack. Avocado on the bottom, cheese in the middle, trout on top—this layering works well and is easy to handle. You can also switch the cheese and trout so that the trout is in the middle. If you are feeling creative, put another slice of avocado on the top for a four-tier effect (plus extra avocado, which is terribly good for you.)

Devilled Eggs

These are a healthy and very Southern treat. It really only requires the cook to be able to boil an egg. Or in this case, a dozen of them.

Ingredients:

1 dozen eggs, boiled
¼ C mayonnaise
1 T prepared mustard
2 T chopped dill pickles (some folks use sweet pickles but I don't hold with that)
Salt and pepper to taste
Ground paprika, as garnish

Boil the eggs and allow them to cool. Peel away the shells and split each egg in half, lengthways. Remove the yolks and put them in a bowl. Arrange the egg whites on a dish. With a fork, mash the yolks until smooth and add in the mayonnaise, mustard and pickles. Continue stirring until this filling is smooth. Add salt and pepper to your taste preference. Stuff the eggs with the yolk filling and sprinkle paprika on the top. Once you've mastered this simple recipe, you'll want to play around with other additions. Finely chopped onion or shallot, a bit of sour cream or yoghurt, capers. Go ahead and try sweet pickle relish, too, if you're feeling brave.

How to Make Butter

Ingredients:

1 C heavy cream (organic, raw if you can get it)
A bit of salt

Put a quart-sized glass canning jar in the fridge. And keep the cream in there, too. When both are thoroughly chilled, pour the cream into the jar, add a little salt and screw the lid on tightly. Put on some dance music and shake the jar until the cream thickens into butter. You will feel the liquid become more and more solid. When it is firm, use a soft spatula to take out the butter and place it in container with a lid and return it to the refrigerator. Then you return to your dancing and have some crispy toast with butter later. Maybe with coffee.

I'm including the following two recipes because they appear in the book. I do not recommend them for a low-fat or low-carb or low-anything diet.

~~~~~~

BARBARA'S BETTER THAN SEX CAKE

Ingredients:

1 C all-purpose flour
1/2 C sweet butter, softened
1 C chopped pecans
1 C powdered sugar
6 ounces of instant chocolate pudding
3 C milk
2—8 ounce tubs of Cool Whip
8 ounces of cream cheese
6 ounces of instant vanilla pudding
1 large chocolate bar

Mix flour, butter and pecans. Press into a 9 x 13 pan. Bake 15 minutes at 350 and allow to cool completely. Mix cream cheese and powdered sugar in a large bowl until fluffy; fold in one tub of Cool Whip. Spread mixture over cooled crust. Combine pudding mixes with three cups of milk until well blended and thick. Spread over cream cheese layer. Spread remaining tub of Cool Whip over pudding layer. Chill overnight and garnish with shaved chocolate. Cut into squares to serve. Or eat with a spoon directly from the pan.

IRENE'S CHERRY YUM YUM

Ingredients:

3 C graham cracker crumbs
1 1/2 sticks sweet butter
8 oz cream cheese
2 pkgs Dream Whip
1 C cold milk
3/4 C sugar
2 cans of cherry pie filling

Mix melted butter and crumbs in a long Pyrex dish. Use a little more than half the crumbs. Press in bottom of dish. Beat Dream Whip and milk. Mix cream cheese and sugar together. Add to Dream Whip mixture. Put half of whip mixture on crust. Spread a layer of cherries on that. Put on rest of whip mixture, then layer on remaining crumbs. Leave in fridge overnight. Serves many, many people.

SUGGESTED READING

A Spy in the House of Love, Anais Nin

Calendar Girl, Audrey Carlan

Delta of Venus, Anais Nin

Herotica, and any of her Anthologies, Susie Bright

Lady Chatterley's Lover, D. H. Lawrence

Little Birds, Anais Nin

Lord of Devil Isle, Connie Mason

Love on a Spoon, C. Margery Kempe

Narcissus in Chains, Laurell K. Hamilton

New Menopausal Years: Alternative Approaches for Women 30-90. Susun Weed

Romance, RR Rose Carbinela

Sacred Selfishness, Masimilla and Bud Harris

Sex and Cupcakes: A Juicy Collection of Essays, Rachel Kramer Bussel

Sleeping Beauty Quartet, Anne Roquelaure

The Boss, Abigail Barnette

The Ravishing of Lady May, Charlotte Lovejoy

The Story of O, Pauline Reage

The Three Rivers, Roberta Latow

Tipping the Velvet, Sarah Waters

Written on the Body, Jeanette Winterson

ABOUT THE AUTHOR

H. Byron Ballard, BA, MFA, is a ritualist, teacher, gardener, speaker and writer. She has served as a featured speaker and teacher at Sacred Space Conference, Pagan Unity Festival, Pagan Spirit Gathering, Southeast Wise Women's Herbal Conference, Glastonbury Goddess Conference, Scottish Pagan Federation Conference, Awakening Our Tribe: CUUPS Convocation and other gatherings.

She is one of the founders and serves as elder priestess at Mother Grove Goddess Temple, a church devoted to the many faces of the Divine Feminine, where she teaches religious education, as well as leads rituals. She is one of the founders of the Coalition of Earth Religions/CERES, a Pagan nonprofit and does interfaith work locally and regionally.

Her writings have appeared in print and electronic media. Her essays are featured in several anthologies and include "Birthed from Scorched Hearts" (Fulcrum Press), "Christmas Presence" (Catawba Press), "Women's Voices in Magic" (Megalithica Books), "Into the Great Below" and "Skalded Apples" (both from Asphodel Press). She blogs as "Asheville's Village Witch" (myvillagewitch.com) and writes as The Village Witch for *Witches and Pagans Magazine* (witchesandPagans.com/The-Village-Witch), where she is also a regular columnist.

Her pamphlet "Back to the Garden: a Handbook for New Pagans" has been widely distributed and she has two books on Appalachian folk magic. *Staubs and Ditchwater: an Introduction to Hillfolks Hoodoo* (Silver Rings Press) and *Asfidity and Mad-Stones* (Smith Bridge Press). Byron is currently at work on *Gnarled Talisman: Old Wild Magics of the Motherlands.* Contact her at www.myvillagewitch.com, info@myvillagewitch.com.

NOTES

NOTES